IBS
FREE AT LAST!

This publication contains the opinions and ideas of its author. It is intended to provide helpful and informative material on how certain individuals can minimize IBS symptoms by manipulating dietary carbohydrates. It is sold with the understanding that the author is not engaged in rendering medical, health or any other kind of personal or professional services. Readers are advised to share the information in this book with a health care provider before adopting any of the suggestions. Readers are advised to discuss symptoms with a medical adviser and not use this book to self-diagnose IBS.

The author and publisher specifically disclaim all responsibility for any liability, loss, or risk, personal or otherwise, incurred as a consequence, directly or indirectly, from the use and application of any of the contents of this book.

ISBN: 0-9820635-0-4
ISBN-13: 9780982063507

Visit www.booksurge.com to order additional copies.

IBS
FREE AT LAST!

The Revolutionary, New Step-by-Step Method
for Those Who Have Tried Everything.

Control IBS symptoms by Limiting FODMAPS
Carbohydrates in Your Diet.

Patsy Catsos, MS, RD, LD
www.ibsfree.net

This book is dedicated to my patients;
it is my great pleasure to know each of you
and my honor to work with you
toward your good health.

Contents

A Personal Note From Patsy Catsos

I WAS 22 YEARS OLD and a dietetic intern at Beth Israel Hospital in Boston, when I presented my first case study of a patient, whose name and face I still recall, with ulcerative colitis. As I studied and wrote about the diagnosis and treatment of bowel disorders, little did I know that I, too, was about to be diagnosed with ulcerative colitis.

Twenty-five years later, I have learned much about gastrointestinal disorders—both as a patient and as a health-care worker who sees patients with bowel conditions. For me, as patient, there have been good years and bad. I have had enough bad years to deeply empathize with my patients suffering from the painful and disabling symptoms of Irritable Bowel Syndrome (IBS). Fortunately, I have been in remission from my colitis for a number of years, although I do experience IBS symptoms when I become careless with my diet.

IBS also takes an emotional toll. I even feel hesitant now, as I sit down to talk briefly about my own challenges and health problems. How will readers react? Will my symptoms be taken seriously? It is hard to put to rest the stereotypes and judgment that IBS sufferers endure every day. People all too often suffer in silence because of social stigmas and the ignorance of others.

I understand how embarrassing it can be to discuss symptoms, even with a physician, family members or friends. I have experienced many of the same awkward moments and difficult social situations that my patients tell me about during our nutrition therapy sessions. I hope this book will offer fellow sufferers some comfort and self-confidence. There are millions of other people out there who share your symptoms and plight.

It has been my personal and professional mission to follow developments in the field of nutrition and gastrointestinal health. While many impressive pharmaceuticals have been researched and marketed, there has been less research devoted to the effects -- both good and bad -- of diet and nutrition. But that seems to be changing, as the medical field comes to grips with an epidemic of obesity as well as GI disorders that cannot be remedied by taking a pill.

IBS sufferers know from firsthand experience that the foods they eat influence symptoms. This book is another step to help patients understand the critical link between diet and IBS. My hope is that this book will enable readers to gain insight into their own eating habits and how they may affect their physical health. Most important, my aim is to help those like myself be free of IBS symptoms.

Preface

THIS BOOK DESCRIBES a step-by-step method for liberating yourself from Irritable Bowel Syndrome (IBS) symptoms triggered by certain dietary carbohydrates. You will start by eating a basic diet containing almost none of these suspect carbohydrates. If the diet is going to help you, you should start to feel better right away, typically within two weeks. After you start feeling better, you will systematically add back one class of carbohydrate foods at a time. By paying attention to your symptoms, you will learn which foods are triggers for your IBS, so that you can limit or avoid them.

In October 2007, I heard the term "FODMAPS" for the first time. A Harvard Medical School professor speaking at a Crohn's and Colitis Foundation of America symposium mentioned in passing that she believed FODMAPS carbohydrates were an important cause of IBS in the United States today. That really caught my ear. Why had I never heard this term before? As a registered, licensed dietitian specializing in the treatment of gastrointestinal disorders and a patient with ulcerative colitis myself, I am certainly well aware of the havoc that IBS symptoms cause in the lives of approximately 15–20 percent of Americans.[1] Here was a new idea that might help my patients. FODMAPS is the acronym for Fermentable

Oligo-, **D**i- and **M**ono-saccharides **A**nd **P**olyols (see Chapter 8 for a detailed explanation).

I immediately made it my business to track down the source of the term FODMAPS, and read all of the available research papers on the subject. Much of the published material on FODMAPS originated at Box Hill Hospital and Monash University in Australia over the past few years. Dietitians Susan J. Shepherd and Jacqueline S. Barrett, as well as Dr. Peter R. Gibson, have been influential leaders in the field, and originated the use of the term FODMAPS.

FODMAPS elimination diets have been used with great success for IBS patients Down Under, but are virtually unknown in the United States. With excitement, I realized the great potential of the information before me, but days of searching on the Internet did not yield any published guides for consumers explaining how to eliminate FODMAPS from the diet.

To fill this void, I created the FODMAPS Elimination Diet based on the research papers I read. In the research setting, focus has been on removing certain carbohydrates from the diet. Knowing which foods to avoid is all well and good, but my clients need to know what they CAN eat. Happily, as I developed the lists of allowed foods for the basic diet, I found they are readily available, nutritious and already present in the cupboards and refrigerators of many people. Without hesitation, I began offering the diet to some of my IBS clients.

If you suffer from IBS, you may not be surprised to hear that some of my clients cried tears of relief mingled with hope as they learned about FODMAPS carbohydrates and how they can cause IBS symptoms. Many were relieved to hear that there might be a reasonable explanation for the failure of their IBS symptoms to respond to conventional therapy. At last, there might be a pain-free way for them to lose weight on a healthy diet. Before these clients left my office, they were showing optimism about the possibility of feeling better in just two weeks.

On the whole, results for my clients in the year since I have been teaching this elimination diet have been outstanding. They come for their follow-up visits with smiles on their faces. After two to three weeks, most tell me they are feeling much, much better. They have more energy and tell me that their bloating, cramping and diarrhea are much improved or almost gone. Sometimes it is not just their IBS symptoms, but other symptoms (such as gastroesophageal reflux disease) that improve with the new way of eating.

A few clients have not experienced much improvement in their symptoms. That is to be expected, since not all cases of IBS involve intolerance to FODMAPS. At least there is some value in ruling out FODMAPS intolerance as a factor in such cases.

Given the promise of these early results, I see no reason to wait any longer before sharing the FODMAPS Elimination Diet with others who may benefit from it. I know there are many of you who will find it life-changing. Although it is based on the latest medical research, as you will see, the diet consists of familiar foods. The diet is safe for healthy individuals, and you will be able to meet all of your nutrient needs with proper planning. If you have other health problems, in addition to IBS, please share the information in the book with your physician or a registered dietitian and ask for help. You may need to modify the food lists to make them medically appropriate for you.

How to Use This Book

This book was written with the non-medically trained reader in mind. Most will benefit from reading the introductory material in Chapters 1–3 to get acquainted with the vocabulary and the ideas behind the diet. There are a few big words to learn, but you soon will become familiar with the most important terms.

If time is short and you already have a firm diagnosis of IBS, it is possible to begin with Chapter 4, which contains a step-by-step method for using the basic diet, including menus, shopping tips and lists of allowed foods. Chapter 5 leads you through the Challenge Phase of the diet. Chapter 6 briefly presents an alternate approach to using the concepts in the book.

Those with an interest in understanding some of the science behind the FODMAPS Elimination Diet will learn much more about carbohydrates and malabsorption in Chapters 7 and 8, which contain slightly more technical reading about carbohydrate malabsorption and FODMAPS. These chapters also will be an excellent review for those with a medical background.

Readers, I look forward to your feedback, which will help me as well as your fellow IBS sufferers. Please visit the web log about this diet, *www.ibsfree.net*, and email me at *patsycatsos@gmail.com*. Let me know how this book has helped you. Send me your questions, so I can address them on my blog and in future editions of this book. I am considering creation of a cookbook for people using the FODMAPS Elimination Diet, and I invite you to send your favorite FODMAPS-friendly recipes.

FODMAPS Elimination Diet Method

Educate yourself about FODMAPS, consult your
physician and get ready (Steps 1, 2, 3, 4)

////

Record your baseline symptoms (Step 5)

////

Plan your diet and go shopping (Steps 6, 7)

////

Eliminate FODMAPS from your diet for at least two weeks;
record symptoms (Steps 8, 9)

////

Evaluate your results compared to baseline;
plan your challenge phase (Step 10)

////

Reintroduce FODMAPS in a series of controlled
challenges; record symptoms (Steps 11, 12, 13, 14)

////

Evaluate results and modify your diet accordingly
(Step 15)
Steps 1–15 are explained in detail in
Chapters 4 and 5
of this book.

Chapter 1
Introduction

Could This Be You?

CLAUDIA, A 52-YEAR-OLD woman, is about 30 pounds overweight and gaining. She has a history of "stomach problems" that goes back to childhood. They seem to be getting worse as she gets older. She experiences bloating and stomach cramps almost every day, and sometimes has explosive diarrhea. She has been seen by a gastroenterology specialist, who diagnosed her with gastroesophageal reflux disease (GERD), but finds nothing that can explain her diarrhea. He tells her it would help her GERD if she lost some weight. But every time she tries to eat healthier—more fruits, veggies, milk and whole grains—she is in so much pain that she feels she must go back to her bad, old ways. Why does eating right have to hurt so much? It doesn't make sense.

Mark was diagnosed with ulcerative colitis at age 25. Now 47, he has suffered for years with uncomfortable symptoms, such as gas, bloating and distressingly urgent diarrhea. He always has blamed these symptoms on the ulcerative colitis, but his recent colonoscopy indicated that his disease is in complete remission. The urgent diarrhea is his biggest problem, making it difficult to leave the house, for fear of not making it to the bathroom in time.

Cathy, age 28, is underweight. She is very health-conscious, and makes a point of getting plenty of fiber in her diet. Cathy has put considerable effort into trying to figure out which foods are triggers for her IBS symptoms (constipation alternating with diarrhea) using a food and symptom diary. It is very confusing to her. It seems she can tolerate certain foods, like yogurt, just fine on one day, but not the next. She has cut so many foods out of her diet that meal planning is difficult and she finds it hard to keep her weight up.

Karin is 16 years old and has such severe IBS symptoms that she sometimes has to stay home from school. The bloating and pain she experiences on a daily basis are limiting her social life. She doesn't dare go out to eat with anyone, and can't travel anywhere her safe foods might not be available. So far, the thing that has helped the most is eliminating milk from her diet. She eats a bland diet, hoping to minimize symptoms, and relies a lot on white bread, pasta and applesauce.

If you can identify with any of these individuals, or parts of their stories, this book is for you.

Eating Well Does Not Have to Hurt

Like the people just described, you may have been experiencing painful gastrointestinal symptoms for years. You may have tried all of the conventional advice, with either no relief or actual worsening of your symptoms. The conventional advice to address your GI symptoms by eating more fiber, fruits, vegetables and whole grains does not work for you. It makes you feel uncomfortable or sick. You already have come to the conclusion that "one size does not fit all."

You may be underweight. Realizing that your symptoms are somehow related to food, but not quite sure how, you may have restricted your diet to the point where you do not get enough variety or enough to eat.

You may be overweight. Many people with IBS tend to limit fruit, vegetables and milk in their diets to avoid symptoms. This leaves the American staples of meat, cheese and every variety of white bread and potatoes. This high-calorie, low-nutrient density diet, consumed in a filling quantity, is enough to make anyone overweight, and certainly does not promote weight loss or good health.

A few of you, especially those prone to constipation, may have noticed that bread just does not agree with you, "stops you right up," and causes gas and bloating. Have you wondered if you might have celiac disease or gluten intolerance? If that has been ruled out by your physician, you will be interested to know that gluten (a protein) is not the only part of wheat that can cause GI problems. Wheat also contains a type of carbohydrate that can cause chaos within your body. You will learn more about that in the pages ahead.

For now, take hope that the elimination diet described within these pages may help you discover a way to eat that is nutritious, safe and painless.

Quiz—Is This Diet for You?

If you answer "yes" to most or all of the following questions, there is an excellent chance that the FODMAPS Elimination Diet will help you:

- 🦶 Have you been diagnosed with IBS, <u>or</u> do you have diarrhea, constipation, gas or bloating that cannot be explained by any other illness or condition?

- Have you already tried the standard dietary advice to increase fiber intake and found it either did not help your IBS symptoms or made you feel worse?

- Have you given up on eating more whole grains, milk, fruits and vegetables because they worsen your IBS symptoms?

- Do you believe your symptoms are related to your diet but find you cannot pin down which foods or beverages are triggers?

- Is your reaction to certain foods inconsistent?

- Have you resigned yourself to living with your symptoms?

- Have you ever had a positive hydrogen breath test for carbohydrate malabsorption?

There is ample evidence that diets limiting FODMAPS carbohydrates can reduce symptoms for IBS patients.[2][3][4][5][6] The FODMAPS Elimination Diet in this book is based on those research findings, although the diet in the format presented here has not been scientifically validated.

A Dietitian Can Help You Set Priorities

You may be asking yourself how this new idea, the FODMAPS Elimination Diet, will fit in with your other dietary priorities. If you are like many of my clients, you may feel overwhelmed at times by too much information and too many competing priorities.

Nutrition advice is beyond abundant. More than 8,000 nutrition-related research papers are published every year.[7] Many of them generate stories in the popular press. The more confusing and contradictory the story is, the better for selling newspapers, magazines and television shows. I am sure you can think of many nutrition topics that have been in the news lately: caffeine, chocolate, wine, folate, calcium, vitamin D, organic food, genetically-modified food, gluten-free food. Are they good for you? Bad for you? Can you afford them?

Add to that your personal situation. You may have a family to plan meals for, each person with different food preferences. You may have other health conditions, such as high blood pressure, high cholesterol or diabetes.

A consultation with a registered dietitian can be extremely helpful for setting priorities, if you have any health conditions in addition to IBS. Your primary care doctor or specialist may have just a short time to spend with you during a typical appointment. Out of necessity, diet is often addressed only briefly, as he or she considers your overall medical condition and treatment.

Dietitians, on the other hand, are medical nutrition therapists. Dietitians in private practice (and in some other settings) can work with you in depth, sorting through your priorities and planning your diet. One way to find a dietitian with a specialty in gastrointestinal disorders is to ask your gastroenterologist or your primary care physician for a referral. Or, you can visit the web site of the American Dietetic Association at *www.eatright.org* and click on "Find a Nutrition Professional."[8] If you are unable to find a dietitian in your area to work with in person, some dietitians work with clients by telephone or via the Internet.

The first step in the nutrition care process is assessment. Like most dietitians in private practice, I usually spend my first one-hour meeting with new clients getting to know their health, diet and exercise histories. I review medications and symptoms, food preferences, family situation and lifestyle. We establish a plan, which often includes a series of follow-up visits. Over time, I guide them through the process described in this book; we evaluate progress and solve problems, adjusting priorities and goals as needed. The goals of treatment for IBS patients are usually to:

- ✔ Eliminate or greatly reduce painful IBS symptoms of gas, bloating, diarrhea or constipation.

- ✔ Learn which foods are triggers for symptoms, and how to enjoy those foods occasionally and in moderation.

- ✔ Plan a "safe" diet that contributes to other healthcare goals, such as weight loss or managing another illness.

This book is based on recently published scientific information that is not yet widely known in the United States medical community, although it is being extensively used in Australia and New Zealand with great success.[9] Your dietitian is undoubtedly familiar with IBS and its conventional treatment. He or she will be familiar with the diagnosis and treatment of lactose malabsorption (lactose is one of the FODMAPS carbohydrates). That model can be used as the basis for understanding the role that malabsorption of the other FODMAPS plays in causing IBS symptoms. Mention this book to your dietitian when you make your appointment. A quick read will bring the dietitian up to speed, and he or she will be ready to help you set dietary priorities.

Medical nutrition therapy is a covered benefit on many medical insurance plans when it is provided by a registered, licensed dietitian. Call the member benefits number on your insurance card or speak to the benefits manager at your workplace to find out whether your plan includes nutrition therapy. Be sure to mention other nutrition-related health conditions you may have in addition to IBS, such as high cholesterol, hypertension, pre-diabetes or diabetes.

You may not need the assistance of a dietitian if you are in good health except for your IBS symptoms, have seen your physician to rule out other medical reasons for the symptoms, and do not have a lot of competing nutrition priorities to plan for. In that case, you should be able to successfully work through this learning process, using the method outlined in this book.

Chapter 2
IBS—Do You Have It?

IBS STANDS FOR **I**rritable **B**owel **S**yndrome. This condition can be defined as "abdominal pain and discomfort with altered bowel habits in the absence of any other mechanical, inflammatory, or biochemical explanation for these symptoms."[10] IBS itself is not a disease, but a collection of symptoms. IBS is often considered a "diagnosis of exclusion." That means it is usually diagnosed after other gastrointestinal disorders and diseases have been ruled out.

IBS affects up to 20 percent of the population, depending on the criteria used to define it.[11] IBS is more common in women than men, and is often diagnosed between the ages of 30 and 50. It can, and does, affect people in other age groups as well. Symptoms may include:

- Constipation and/or diarrhea
- Gas
- Bloating or abdominal distension
- Abdominal pain relieved by moving your bowels

The origins of IBS are not well understood by clinicians and scientists. Over the years, our view of IBS has changed and evolved and will probably continue to do so. At the present time, it seems likely that IBS arises from some combination of the following:[12] [13]

- Abnormal contraction and relaxation of the intestinal muscles that move food through the gastrointestinal system, known as a *motility disorder*. Motility disorders may cause food to move through the GI tract too slowly or quickly, and can sometimes cause intestinal muscle spasms to occur.

- Low pain threshold for distention in the intestines of affected individuals, known as *visceral hypersensitivity*.[14] This means that a buildup of gas or fluids in the large intestine may hurt the IBS sufferer but not cause a painful sensation to someone who does not have IBS.

- Miscommunication between the gut and the brain, possibly relating to a *nervous system dysfunction*.

Stress and inflammation may influence these three proposed origins of IBS in ways that are unclear at this time.

IBS is sometimes further described based on primary symptoms. It may be described as constipation-predominant, diarrhea-predominant, or pain-predominant.[15] Treatment usually is directed at the most troubling symptoms.

Ruling Out Other Conditions

You should not diagnose yourself with IBS. If you experience symptoms suggestive of IBS, seek a thorough medical evaluation to rule out other potentially serious conditions, especially if you are experiencing any of the following:

- passing blood, pus or mucous from the rectum
- anal or rectal problems such as abscesses, skin tags, fissures or hemorrhoids
- fevers or night sweats
- aching joints or inflammatory arthritis
- anemia or other abnormal lab results
- malnutrition
- unplanned weight loss greater than 10 pounds
- onset of symptoms after age 50
- poor growth or failure to thrive (in children)
- itchy rash or diagnosis of dermatitis herpetiformis
- family history of Crohn's disease, ulcerative colitis, celiac disease, or colon cancer
- foul-smelling, greasy or floating stools
- incontinence or soiling
- urge to move bowels waking you from sleep
- osteoporosis or osteopenia
- thyroid dysfunction

Your health care provider will consider the pattern of your symptoms and compare them to established criteria. He or she will take into account your medical and family history, a physical examination, and the results of appropriate tests. In younger patients without "alarm symptoms,"[16] a limited work-up may be sufficient to diagnose IBS.

Once you have a reasonably firm diagnosis of IBS, you can begin the FODMAPS Elimination Diet with confidence.

IBS in Combination with Other GI Disorders

It is not unusual to have IBS, in addition to another GI problem, such as Crohn's disease or ulcerative colitis. In fact, a third of those individuals with ulcerative colitis and over half of those with Crohn's also have IBS.[17] During flare-ups, FODMAPS can be poorly tolerated and add misery to your symptoms.

Crohn's or ulcerative colitis patients sometimes experience gas, bloating, diarrhea or constipation even when they are technically in remission (no active inflammation). If you have Crohn's or colitis, you may be able to experience further relief of symptoms during remission by using the FODMAPS Elimination Diet.[18] [19] During flare-ups, the diet may help control symptoms while allowing you to eat a diet rich in healing nutrients.

Many of my overweight patients have gastroesophageal reflux disease (GERD) or Barrett's esophagus, in addition to IBS. While using the FODMAPS Elimination Diet to treat IBS, some of them have experienced remarkable improvement in their GERD symptoms as well.

My point is this: If you are being treated for another GI disorder but are still symptomatic, some further improvement in your symptoms may be possible with the use of the FOD-MAPS Elimination Diet. I advise you to discuss the possibility with your gastroenterologist.

Difference Between IBS and IBD

IBD stands for **I**nflammatory **B**owel **D**isease, and should not be confused with IBS. Inflammatory bowel diseases include Crohn's disease and ulcerative colitis. Unlike IBS, IBD causes significant inflammation, ulcers and other damage to the gastrointestinal tract. To arrive at a diagnosis of irritable bowel syndrome, your physician will first make sure you do not have IBD, which is more serious and requires different medical management.

A Note About Celiac Disease

Because part of the FODMAPS diet involves temporarily eliminating wheat products, the subject of celiac disease is bound to come up, and needs some clarification.

Celiac disease, also known as celiac sprue or gluten intolerance, results from intolerance to a *protein (gluten)* present in wheat, barley and rye. Wheat in any amount is toxic to someone with celiac disease, and should never be deliberately consumed by sufferers.

On the other hand, on the FODMAPS Elimination Diet, the focus is on the type of *carbohydrate* found in wheat. Eating wheat products does not cause physical damage to the intestines of the IBS sufferer, as it does to the individual with celiac disease. As long as you don't also have celiac disease (or a wheat allergy), after the initial elimination phase of this diet, wheat can be eaten in small amounts, or as much as you find you can tolerate.

Tests for celiac disease are only accurate if you have been eating a diet that includes plenty of gluten. A wheat-free diet could cause tests to come back with "false negative" results. If your doctor plans to test you for celiac disease, make arrangements to have it done before starting the FODMAPS Elimination Diet.

Who Should NOT Use This Diet Without Modification

While the FODMAPS Elimination Diet should be safe for most individuals, there are some situations that require modification of the diet. Please consult a registered dietitian for assistance if you have

- Hereditary Fructose Intolerance (HFI)

- Food allergies

- Been diagnosed with any medical conditions that have special dietary needs or that require the use of prescription medications

Hereditary Fructose Intolerance

Hereditary fructose intolerance (HFI) is a condition that deserves special mention. Fructose is one of the FODMAPS carbohydrates. There is a big difference between fructose *malabsorption*, which can cause IBS symptoms to occur, and *hereditary fructose intolerance.* To further clarify the terminology, the collection of symptoms resulting from fructose malabsorption is sometimes referred to as *dietary* (as opposed to hereditary) fructose intolerance.

HFI is an inborn error of metabolism, and individuals with this disorder cannot and should not consume any fructose at all, no matter how small the amount. Many individuals with HFI are diagnosed in infancy or childhood, when caregivers note the child is violently ill after ingesting anything containing fructose, such as table sugar or honey. Some adults have undiagnosed HFI; they have an absolute aversion to sweets of any kind, going back to childhood. This "dislike" of sweets may run in the family. If you have HFI or suspect you may have HFI, there are some foods on the elimination diet that you should not consume. Please consult a dietitian before proceeding with the diet.

Food Allergies

Food allergies are another condition requiring modification of the diet. Foods consist of many components, not just the carbohydrates this diet focuses on. There may be foods on the "allowed" lists, or foods that are on the "challenge" lists that you should not eat because you are allergic to the protein component of the foods. Before embarking on the diet, take out a pen and cross out any foods to which you are allergic. If you have a diagnosed allergy to any food, you should NEVER add it back to your diet or challenge yourself with the food without medical supervision.

There may be foods that you aren't actually allergic to, but which have caused discomfort for you in the past. For example, corn and lettuce do not contain large amounts of FODMAPS, so they are "allowed" foods on the diet. They do, however, contain a lot of insoluble fiber, and many of my clients report these foods are poorly digested, even visible and unchanged in their stool. While this could be remedied somewhat by thorough and careful chewing of each mouthful of food, feel free to avoid items on the food lists that cause you distress for any reason. You always can try adding them back at another time to test your tolerance.

Medical Conditions

Finally, if you have another medical condition that has dietary implications, you should seek special help from a registered dietitian to make sure that you do not consume any foods during the elimination phase or the challenge phase that are harmful or will worsen your condition. Examples of these conditions are *gout, gastroesophageal reflux, kidney stones, gastroparesis, diverticulitis, and celiac disease.* Examples of medications that require extra care with the diet are *insulin, warfarin* (Coumadin), and *cholesterol-lowering medications* such as Lipitor. This list is not exhaustive. If you are not sure whether one of your medical conditions or medications requires you to avoid certain foods, please consult your health care provider.

Standard Therapy for IBS

This section briefly touches upon a number of standard therapies for IBS, which have been discussed in great detail in many other publications. It is assumed that IBS sufferers who are reading this book are familiar with, and have tried, standard therapies for IBS. If the treatments mentioned in this section do not sound familiar to you, please take the time to explore them. Although pursuing the FODMAPS Elimination Diet is unlikely to do any harm, it is possible that something simpler, such as increasing your fiber or fluid intake, may improve your symptoms.

Therapy for IBS depends on which symptoms predominate, and how severe they are. For all types, stress management, exercise, and use of various medications (ranging from anti-spasmodics to anti-diarrheals to anti-depressants) may help.[20][21] Use of probiotics, or stocking the gut with beneficial bacteria, is often recommended for those with IBS.

Individuals with constipation-predominate IBS are often counseled to increase fiber intake from foods such as whole grains, fruits and vegetables. Many people use fiber supplements to boost their fiber intake. Regular exercise and drinking plenty of fluids can also be helpful in the treatment of constipation. These measures help many people manage constipation, and should be tried first.

Those with diarrhea-predominant IBS often are advised to avoid milk products, caffeine, "gassy" foods, and non-nutritive fats, such as those in fat-free potato chips. Ice cold and steaming hot beverages may be avoided. "Safe" foods for diarrhea-predominant IBS have traditionally included pasta, white bread, applesauce, and yogurt. Dietary fiber and fiber supplements are often recommended for diarrhea, not just constipation. To prevent watery stools, soluble fiber is sometimes able to "gel" the intestinal contents. If these measures help, good for you. If not, read on.

The FODMAPS Elimination Diet is meant for people who have tried standard therapies for IBS but have failed to find relief from their symptoms. Many IBS sufferers stick with conventional therapies for years without noticeable results, and become resigned to their symptoms.

In fact, my clients often do not seek medical nutrition therapy for IBS alone. More often, clients seek treatment because they are overweight, which may be causing difficulties with blood pressure, high cholesterol, or blood sugar. When I hear that they have never been able to lose weight because "healthy foods" cause bloating, gas, constipation or diarrhea, I know that I have met another candidate for the FODMAPS Elimination Diet. Other clients may begin treatment because they are underweight. Progress can begin toward weight gain, weight loss or other health-care goals once disruptive IBS symptoms have been tamed.

Chapter 3
FODMAPS Elimination Diet FAQs

What are FODMAPS?

O_{K, I KNOW} I promised to keep this in layman's terms, but here comes an awkward paragraph with some new vocabulary. Stay with me, though, because you won't want to miss the rest of this chapter. It will help you understand how the FODMAPS Elimination Diet works.

The diet is based on limiting "FODMAPS" in the diet. FODMAPS stands for **F**ermentable **O**ligo-, **D**i- and **M**onosaccharides **A**nd **P**olyols. Specifically, some of the dietary carbohydrates described by the term FODMAPS are lactose, fructose, fructans, polyols and galactans. Don't worry about remembering all of these terms. It's more important to understand that all of the FODMAPS have several things in common.

FODMAPS carbohydrates are sugars, starches and fibers in food that some people cannot fully digest and absorb. This is called *malabsorption*. FODMAPS are found in certain grains, fruits, vegetables, dried peas and beans, milk products and prepared foods and beverages. In some people, ingested FODMAPS carbohydrates are not absorbed as they should be in the small intestine; instead they pass into the large intestine. Humans have large numbers of bacteria living in the large intestine. This is normal. The problem is that FOD-MAPS act as "fast food" for the bacteria, which give off a lot of gas as they ferment the food.[22] The gas makes your large intestine bloat (swell). If you have IBS, your intestines may be extra sensitive to this, and it hurts. It may cause constipation or diarrhea.

Another problem with FODMAPS is the way they pull water into your large intestine. This is called *osmosis*. One way to imagine osmosis is to picture what happens when you sprinkle sugar on freshly cut strawberries. The sugar attracts the water from the strawberries to itself. The sugar pulls the juice right out of the strawberries and into the bowl. In your large intestine, FODMAPS pull water out of your cells and into your large intestine in the same manner, causing it to bloat. Pain and watery diarrhea can result.

All FODMAPS are believed to cause IBS symptoms the same way: too much gas and water in your large intestine. It is hard to figure out what foods are causing the problem, unless you look at the big picture and take into account all five different kinds of FODMAPS at the same time. All five get thrown into the same "bucket." If you eat too much of them, they may overflow into the large intestine. The effects are cumulative; the more FODMAPS you eat in one day, the worse your symptoms are likely to be.[23]

That is why you may be able to get away with eating ice cream or bread one day but not on another. On the "bad" day, you may have eaten a lot of other FODMAPS carbohydrate foods without realizing it. Until now, this has made it very difficult to identify which foods are causing your IBS symptoms.

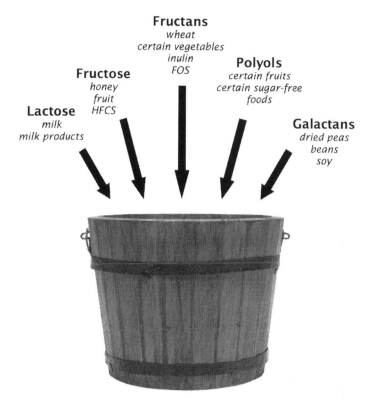

Fructans
wheat
certain vegetables
inulin
FOS

Fructose
honey
fruit
HFCS

Lactose
milk
milk products

Polyols
certain fruits
certain sugar-free
foods

Galactans
dried peas
beans
soy

All dietary FODMAPS go into the same "bucket."

The bucket represents your unique, personal capacity to tolerate FODMAPS carbohydrates from all sources. If your FODMAPS intake exceeds your capacity for digestion and absorbtion in the small intestine, overflow into the large intestine occurs. This may result in IBS symptoms in sensitive individuals.

It is the total volume of gas and water produced by your gut bacteria from all FODMAPS sources that causes the problem. The offending FODMAPS may be from a large quantity of one food or smaller amounts of several different foods added together.

Why Do FODMAPS Cause IBS Symptoms for Some People and Not for Others?

There are a number of factors that may explain why FODMAPS cause more troublesome symptoms for some people than for others. For example, individuals vary a great deal in how much lactase they produce, with half or more of adults having reduced lactase activity.[24]

Lactase is the enzyme needed to digest the milk sugar lactose, which is one of the FODMAPS carbohydrates. Without it, undigested milk sugar is presented to the bacteria in the large intestine, where it acts as a source of food for them. Even lactase-deficient people can usually tolerate small amounts of lactose in the diet (up to 7 grams in one sitting).[25] In combination with the other FODMAPS, however, smaller amounts may cause difficulty.

Fructose absorption also varies widely from one person to the next. For reasons that are not clear, up to one half of the adult population may malabsorb fructose.[26][27][28] Also, the amount of other sugars, sugar alcohols, and certain amino acids in the meal affect how completely fructose is absorbed. It appears to be normal for humans to malabsorb fructose to some extent, especially if a large amount of fructose has been consumed.[29] Unabsorbed fructose that is delivered to the large intestine can cause chaos when it is digested by the resident bacteria.

Likewise, it is normal for fructans (found in wheat and some fruits and vegetables) and galactans (found in beans and some vegetables) to be almost entirely malabsorbed in all people. Being essentially indigestible is part of what defines fructans and galactans as fiber.

People with more adaptable bowels are not bothered by symptoms when consuming these foods unless they eat an unusually large portion, and may in fact use these foods deliberately to "stay regular." As the saying goes, "one man's meat is another man's poison." Those with less adaptable bowels may experience IBS symptoms after consuming these foods. In some individuals the nervous system serving the gut is more sensitive and responds with pain to gut distention.

On another note, some individuals have such a fast intestinal transit time that FODMAPS do not have a chance to be absorbed before being presented to the bacteria in the large intestine. Others have slow intestinal transit time. There is some evidence that constipation is associated with the presence of methane in the breath of affected individuals.[30] Breath methane would likely be the result of methane-producing bacteria in the large intestine. It is not clear yet what this means, but it may somehow influence why some people with IBS have constipation and others do not.

Finally, some individuals have bacteria inappropriately growing in the small intestine that start fermenting FODMAPS before they can be absorbed.[31] The sooner IBS symptoms occur after eating, the greater the possibility of small intestine bacterial overgrowth (SIBO). The role of SIBO in IBS is intriguing but still unclear.[32]

Some or all of the above factors may cause IBS symptoms in a single person. The FODMAPS Elimination Diet has the potential to improve symptoms caused by all of them, by depriving the gut bacteria of their favorite foods: undigested sugars and complex carbohydrates.

Why is This Method Called an Elimination Diet?

This is not necessarily a diet to stay on for life. It is a diet for learning—essentially an experiment, with you as the subject. The diet is designed to help you figure out whether you are sensitive to FODMAPS carbohydrates, and which ones are causing your symptoms. This type of diet is sometimes called an *elimination diet*. Just as the term describes, an elimination diet eliminates foods that are suspected of causing symptoms in a person with IBS.

The basic diet is the most restrictive, with all foods high in FODMAPS eliminated. If your IBS symptoms are caused by FODMAPS carbohydrates, you will typically experience a positive response within the first two weeks after eliminating them. Don't worry; you do not have to give up all of the FODMAPS-containing foods forever. In the next steps of the process, called the *challenge phase*, you will challenge yourself with each class of FODMAPS carbohydrates, one class at a time, by returning foods to your diet in a controlled way. In this way you will learn which FODMAPS you can tolerate and in what amounts.

At the end of the challenge phase, you will have the ability to choose the most liberal diet you can tolerate. You can decide on a given day whether you want to "pay the price" of splurging on a particular type or amount of food. Or, you can modify your intake of other FODMAPS that day to minimize symptoms. It is up to you, once you are in control.

What About Other Treatments for IBS During the Diet?

At the end of the previous chapter, you read a brief summary of standard therapy for IBS. Perhaps you have tried many of these approaches. While you are experimenting with the FODMAPS Elimination Diet, you can continue any of these practices that seem to be helping you. If you stop or start any of these practices in the middle of your experiment, it may cause confusion as you try to interpret the results. In particular, you should not stop taking medications that have been prescribed for you without consulting your physician.

To maximize the learning value of the FODMAPS Elimination Diet, keep the rest of your routine consistent throughout the diet. Then, if your symptoms improve, you will know the change in your diet was the cause.

How Long Does it Take to Get Results?

You begin by eliminating all significant sources of FODMAPS carbohydrates in the diet. If FODMAPS foods are the triggers for your IBS symptoms, your symptoms will improve quickly, as a rule within two weeks.

You can stay with the elimination phase for as long as you like. It is entirely possible to select a varied and nutritious diet from the "allowed" foods on the diet. I have clients who are feeling so good on the elimination phase that they have not wanted to rock the boat by embarking on the challenge phase.

If you choose to, you can march through the challenge phase in 6 weeks or so. Or you can stretch it out over as much time as you like.

How Will I Know if it Worked?

The best way to know if the elimination diet worked is to keep accurate records. Before you start the diet, use a symptom rating worksheet (see Appendix) to keep track of your IBS symptoms for a whole week while eating your usual diet. This will be your baseline symptom profile. During the elimination phase, in other words your first two weeks on the basic diet, continue to rate your IBS symptoms. If the FODMAPS elimination is working, there should be a sharp drop in the number and type of symptoms you experience by the end of the second week. Studying these numbers and comparing them to your baseline symptoms will help you decide whether the diet worked, and which classes of carbohydrates are triggers for you. You will be the one who ultimately decides whether the diet is right for you and whether FODMAPS carbohydrates are the source of your IBS symptoms.

What if the Diet Does Not Work?

It is a fact that for some individuals, IBS symptoms may not be triggered by FODMAPS carbohydrate malabsorption. Even this information can be a valuable outcome of the elimination diet. You'll be free to enjoy foods knowing that they are probably not IBS triggers for you, at least not because they contain FODMAPS.

Note that some scientists and clinicians have found that foods can trigger IBS symptoms in certain individuals by another mechanism: *delayed immune response.* The program that has been developed to treat this is called LEAP therapy. LEAP stands for Lifestyle Eating and Performance. The program uses a procedure patented by Signet Diagnostic Corporation (known as Mediator Release Testing) to test blood for sensitivity to a large number of foods and chemicals. A detailed, customized rotation diet is then planned for each patient based on the results of the testing.[33] Specially trained dietitians work with patients throughout the program. Although further discussion of LEAP is outside the scope of this book, you may wish to look into it if you do not experience relief on the FODMAPS Elimination Diet.

Is This a Weight Loss Diet?

No. The FODMAPS Elimination Diet is not meant to be a weight loss diet. The word "diet" is used here in a more general sense, to describe the array of foods and beverages that you are consuming. If you would benefit from gaining or losing weight, you may be much more successful achieving your goals after you have used the FODMAPS Elimination Diet to identify the foods that you can tolerate well.

Can Vegetarians Use This Diet?

Lacto-ovo vegetarians can meet their protein needs on this diet by choosing eggs, cheese, lactose-free milk products, and high-protein whole grains (such as quinoa) each day. Vegans will have a very difficult time getting enough protein on the FODMAPS Elimination Diet, because soy products and other dried peas and beans are not allowed on the basic diet. Vegans can successfully use the alternate approach described in Chapter 6, because it won't be necessary to go without soy, peas and beans for more than a week.

How Does This Method Compare to the Atkins Diet?

The Atkins Diet is a *very* low carbohydrate diet. The FODMAPS Elimination diet is not. Rather, it is a carbohydrate-*controlled* diet, with the major focus on the *type* of carbohydrate. There is no limit on total carbohydrate intake, although intake of some particular sugars and complex carbohydrates is restricted.

Chapter 4
The Elimination Phase

THIS CHAPTER DESCRIBES the elimination phase of this step-by-step method for liberating yourself from IBS symptoms possibly caused by intolerance to certain carbohydrates. You will start by eating a basic diet containing little or none of these suspect carbohydrates. If the diet is going to help you, you should start to feel better right away, typically within two weeks. After you start feeling better, you will systematically add back one class of carbohydrates at a time. By paying attention to your symptoms, you will learn which foods are triggers for your IBS, so that you can limit or avoid them.

The following steps tell you what to do before starting the diet.

Step 1: Consult Your Physician

Have you seen your physician to rule out gastrointestinal diseases or other possible reasons for your gas, bloating, diarrhea, constipation or abdominal pain? Make an appointment with your physician to discuss your symptoms. Do not diagnose yourself with IBS.

Step 2: Consider Your Other Medical Problems

Review the section in Chapter 2 entitled, "Who Should Not Use This Diet Without Modification," to make sure this diet is appropriate for you. If you have any medical problems or take prescription medications, this is a good time to consult with a registered dietitian for assistance.

Review all of the foods listed on the basic diet. **Cross out any foods that you are allergic to, cannot tolerate, or should not eat for any other reason.**

Step 3: Do Not Change the Other Things You Do for IBS

If you take any medications or use any other treatments for IBS, do not change them during the basic phase of the elimination diet. There are two exceptions. One: If you use a bulk fiber laxative, consult your health care provider or check the manufacturer's web site to make sure it does not contain fermentable carbohydrates (FODMAPS). Two: If you use a probiotic supplement that includes FOS (fructo-oligosaccharides), you may want to consider switching to a similar supplement without FOS for the duration of the basic diet, because FOS is a FODMAPS carbohydrate.

Step 4: Choose a Start Date

Choose a start date, at least one week ahead of when you want to start the diet itself. During this time you will rate your baseline symptoms, plan meals and grocery shop (Steps 5, 6 and 7). Write your start date here: _____

Step 5: Rate Your Baseline Symptoms

During the week before your start date, rate your symptoms while eating your usual diet, using a symptom rating worksheet (see Appendix). This will be your baseline symptom profile. If you really cannot wait to start, think back over the week before you read this book and write down your estimated score for each symptom. In your enthusiasm to begin the diet, *please do not skip this step*. Without it, you will not learn as much from this whole process. Trust me on this, once you are feeling better it will not take long to forget how badly you felt just a short time ago.

You will need at least 10 copies of the symptom rating worksheet. You may find it helpful to prepare them at this time.

Step 6: Prepare a Menu from Foods on the Allowed Lists

Consider writing out your menu for the entire first week. If you wish, you can use or adapt the sample menu in this section for your own use. You can then repeat the menu during week two. Using a prepared menu will help you make sure you have enough allowed foods on hand.

It will be easier for you if your menu is relatively simple, and if you prepare most of your own food during the first two weeks of the basic diet. Focus on reading labels and observing your symptoms, not preparing elaborate meals.

Individual calorie needs vary from person to person. The sample menu provided is not meant to promote weight loss or gain, and if either is desired, please consult a registered dietitian for assistance. For the record, the sample menu provides in the neighborhood of 2,000 calories per day, chosen because this calorie level is commonly used as a reference for food labeling and recommendations about nutrient intake. If it seems like too much or too little for you, please adjust accordingly, while imitating the variety and moderation modeled. Those with smaller needs or appetites may wish to eliminate the snacks on the menu.

Take a look at the sample menu provided. It illustrates several important rules for meal planning on the elimination phase:

- On the basic diet, you should eat only foods on the allowed lists and avoid those that are not specifically named on the lists.

- Don't make the common mistake of jumping to the conclusion that one of the categories of FODMAPS is not a problem for you because you eat it routinely. You may be tempted to think that wheat or milk, for example, isn't your problem because you can sometimes consume it without experiencing symptoms. As you now know, this may be the result of having less of the other FODMAPS to eat on those good days. Don't make any assumptions. Don't make exceptions. Eat ONLY foods on the basic diet for best results. It's only for two weeks— you can do it!

- Portion sizes are important for many foods. Foods listed in **bold-face type** must be consumed in limited portions because they do contain small amounts of FODMAPS.

- Consume only one bold-face food per meal or snack, to limit the total FODMAPS load to a very low level, which will be unlikely to provoke any symptoms.

Portion sizes are offered for other foods merely as suggestions, to help answer the question, "What is a good portion size?" You can vary the portions according to your needs and appetite.

Except for the rule to limit yourself to one bold-face food per meal or snack, this plan does not attempt to instruct you on how many servings to eat from each food group. There are too many variables falling outside the scope of this book to consider. Just remember that variety and moderation are the keys to a healthy diet. You may feel much better in just a short time, if you choose fewer empty calories and more nutrient-rich foods. With the FODMAPS Elimination Diet, you may finally be able to eat the fruits, vegetables, whole grains and dairy products your body craves and needs.

A few final comments are needed about the sample menus: There are several variations of the breakfast and morning snack pattern to take into account the various ways that people take their coffee. Since fruit is part of each breakfast, and is bold-face item, if you take cream in your coffee (also a bold-face item) you should hold off on that until snack time. Days with sugar for coffee included at breakfast have fewer Extras later in the day.

Like real life, there is some repetition in the sample menu. If you buy a package of food, say berries, it is assumed you want to use the package up before it goes bad, so you will see it repeated on the menu several times. If you prefer, you can easily make substitutions to the sample menu by consulting the food lists in Step 8. You can also design your own menu from scratch to suit your food preferences.

Recipes used in the sample menu are provided in the Appendix.

⚉ Day 1

BREAKFAST
> 1 cup Cheerios (Grains/Starches)
> 1 cup lactose-free skim milk (Meats/Milk)
> 2 tablespoons chopped walnuts (Fats)
> **½ ripe banana (Fruits)**

MORNING SNACK
> 3 plain rice cakes (Grains/Starches)
> 1 hard boiled egg (Meats/Milk)

LUNCH
> 2 slices wheat-free bread (Grains/Starches)
> 3 ounces turkey (Meats/Milk)
> Lettuce and tomato (Vegetables)
> 2 tablespoons light mayonnaise (Fats)
> **¾ cup blueberries (Fruits)**
> ½ cup baby carrots (Vegetables)

AFTERNOON SNACK
> ½ cup lactose-free cottage cheese (Meats/Milk)
> 8 cherry tomatoes (Vegetables)

DINNER
> ½ medium baked potato (Grains/Starches)
> **1-1/2 tablespoons sour cream (Fats)**
> 4 ounces baked salmon (Meats/Milk)
> 2 cups raw baby spinach (Vegetables)
> 1 cup mixed green peppers and mushrooms (Veg)
> 1 teaspoon olive oil (Fat)
> 1 tablespoon balsamic vinegar
> 4 fluid ounces red wine, optional

EVENING SNACK
> ¼ cup peanuts (Fats)

BEVERAGES
> Water, coffee and/or tea as desired

⚏ Day 2

BREAKFAST

> 1 cup Cheerios (Grains/Starches)
>
> 1 cup lactose-free skim milk (Meats/Milk)
>
> **½ ripe banana (Fruits)**

MORNING SNACK

> 14 small rice crackers (Grains/Starches)
>
> 1 hard boiled egg (Meats/Milk)
>
> **2 tablespoons half-and-half for coffee (Fats)**

LUNCH

> 2 slices wheat-free bread (Grains/Starches)
>
> 3 ounces tuna (Meats/Milk)
>
> 2 tablespoons light mayonnaise (Fats)
>
> Lettuce and tomato (Vegetables)
>
> **1 small orange (Fruits)**
>
> ½ cup baby carrots (Vegetables)

AFTERNOON SNACK

> **1 ounce low-fat mozzarella cheese stick
>   (Meats/Milk)**
>
> 8 cherry tomatoes (Vegetables)

DINNER

> 1 cup brown rice (Grains/Starches)
>
> 4 ounces grilled chicken (Meats/Milk)
>
> 4 cups mixed salad greens (Vegetables)
>
> 2 tablespoons slivered almonds (Fats)
>
> 1 teaspoon olive oil (Fats)
>
> 1 tablespoon balsamic vinegar
>
> **2 peanut butter cookies (Extras-recipe provided)**

EVENING SNACK

> **1 tangerine (Fruits)**

BEVERAGES

> Water, coffee and/or tea as desired

⫴ Day 3

BREAKFAST

    1 cup Cheerios (Grains/Starches)

    1 cup lactose-free skim milk (Meats/Milk)

    2 tablespoons walnuts (Fats)

    1 ½ tablespoons sugar for coffee (Extras)

MORNING SNACK

    ¾ cup blueberries (Fruits)

    ½ cup lactose-free cottage cheese (Meats/Milk)

LUNCH

    1 cup sweet potato, baked (Grains/Starches)

    3 ounces grilled chicken (Meats/Milk)

    1 cup steamed cauliflower/broccoli florets (Veg)

    1 teaspoon margarine (Fats)

    2 peanut butter cookies (Extras—recipes provided)

AFTERNOON SNACK

    1 ounce low-fat mozzarella cheese stick

        (Meats/Milk)

    1 medium bell pepper, strips (Vegetables)

DINNER

    1 cup rice pasta (Grains/Starches)

    4 ounces pork loin (Meats/Milk)

    2 teaspoons canola oil (Fats)

    2 cups mushrooms and carrots, stir fried (Veg)

    Soy sauce, wheat-free (Extras)

    1 tangerine (Fruits)

EVENING SNACK

    2 tablespoons almonds (Fats)

BEVERAGES

    Water, coffee and/or tea as desired

〽 Day 4

BREAKFAST

    1 cup sliced potatoes (Grains/Starches)

    1 egg (Meats/Milk)

    2 teaspoons margarine (Fats)

    1/3 cup orange juice (Fruits)

MORNING SNACK

    ½ cup cooked oatmeal (Grain/Starch)

    1 cup lactose-free skim milk (Meats/Milk)

LUNCH

    2 slices wheat-free bread (Grains/Starches)

    3 ounces turkey (Meats/Milk)

    Lettuce and tomato (Vegetables)

    2 tablespoons light mayonnaise (Fats)

    ¾ cup blueberries (Fruits)

    ½ cup baby carrots (Vegetables)

AFTERNOON SNACK

    ½ cup lactose-free cottage cheese (Meats/Milk)

    1 cup peeled cucumber slices (Vegetables)

DINNER

    2 corn tortillas (Grains/Starches)

    4 ounces grilled steak (Meats/Milk)

    1 cup sautéed green pepper strips (Vegetables)

    2 teaspoons olive oil (Fats)

    ½ cup chopped tomato (Vegetables)

    Tabasco sauce (Extras)

    1 ½ tablespoons sour cream (Fats)

    4 fluid ounces red wine, optional (Extras)

EVENING SNACK

    1 cup strawberries (Fruits)

    ¼ cup almonds (Fats)

BEVERAGES

    Water, coffee and/or tea as desired

⫻ Day 5

BREAKFAST

> 1 cup cooked oatmeal (Grains/Starches)
>
> 1 cup lactose-free skim milk (Meats/Milk)
>
> 2 tablespoons chopped walnuts (Fats)
>
> **½ ripe banana (Fruits)**

MORNING SNACK

> 3 plain rice cakes (Grains/Starches)
>
> **2 ounces low-fat cheese (Meats/Milk)**

LUNCH

> 1 ounce baked potato chips (Grains/Starches)
>
> 4 cups mixed salad greens (Vegetables)
>
> ½ cup mixed cucumber and mushrooms (Veg)
>
> 3 ounces turkey (Meats/Milk)
>
> 1 tablespoon olive oil (Fats)
>
> 2 tablespoons wine vinegar

AFTERNOON SNACK

> ½ cup lactose-free cottage cheese (Meats/Milk)
>
> **¾ cup blueberries (Fruits)**

DINNER

> 1 serving Shepherd's Pie (Grains/Starches, Vegetables,
> Meats/Milk, Fats—recipe provided)
>
> **1 small orange (Fruits)**

EVENING SNACK

> 14 small rice crackers
>
> 1/3 cup peanuts

BEVERAGES

> Water, coffee and/or tea as desired

※ Day 6

BREAKFAST

    1 cup Cheerios (Grains/Starches)

    1 cup lactose-free skim milk (Meats/Milk)

    2 tablespoons chopped walnuts (Fats)

    1 cup strawberries (Fruits)

MORNING SNACK

    14 small rice crackers (Grains/Starches)

    1 hard boiled egg (Meats/Milk)

LUNCH

    1 slice wheat-free toast (Grains/Starches)

    1 teaspoon margarine (Fats)

    1 serving Meatball Soup (Meats/Milk, Vegetables, Grains/Starches—recipe provided)

    ¾ cup blueberries (Fruits)

AFTERNOON SNACK

    1 ounce low-fat cheese (Meats/Milk)

    ½ cup baby carrots (Vegetables)

DINNER

    1 serving Shrimp Pasta Primavera (Grains/Starches, Meats/Milk, Fats, Vegetables—recipe provided)

EVENING SNACK

    ½ ripe banana (Fruits)

    1 tablespoon peanut butter (Fats)

BEVERAGES

    Water, coffee and/or tea as desired

⁄⁄⁄ Day 7

BREAKFAST

    1 cup Cheerios (Grains/Starches)

    1 cup lactose-free skim milk (Meats/Milk)

    2 tablespoons chopped walnuts (Fats)

    1 cup strawberries (Fruits)

MORNING SNACK

    12 small rice crackers (Grain/Starch)

    1 cup lactose-free milk (Meats/Milk)

LUNCH

    1 slice wheat-free bread (Grains/Starches)

    1 teaspoon margarine (Fats)

    1 serving Meatball Soup (Meats/Milk, Vegetables,
        Grains/Starches—recipe provided)

    1/3 cup orange juice (Fruits)

AFTERNOON SNACK

    2 slices lean deli roast beef (Meats/Milk)

    1 medium red bell pepper, strips (Vegetable)

DINNER

    1 cup brown rice (Grains/Starches)

    6 ounces plain grilled chicken (Meats/Milk)

    2 cups mixed salad greens (Vegetables)

    2 tablespoons slivered almonds (Fats)

    1 teaspoon olive oil (Fats)

    1 tablespoon balsamic vinegar

    ½ cup strawberry sorbet, sugar sweetened

EVENING SNACK

    ½ ripe banana (Fruits)

    1 tablespoon peanut butter (Fats)

BEVERAGES

    Water, coffee and/or tea as desired

Step 7: Go Grocery Shopping

A shopping list for the sample menu is provided below. Using a shopping list based on your Week 1 menu will ensure that you have all of your allowed foods on hand, and help your first week go smoothly.

⫸ **Week 1 Shopping List**

Grocery Items

1 box Cheerios

8 ounce box quick oats

8 ounces chopped walnuts

4 ounces slivered almonds

8 ounces whole almonds

1 small jar light mayonnaise

8 fluid ounces olive oil

12 ounce jar creamy peanut butter

8 fluid ounces canola oil

8 fluid ounces balsamic vinegar

.75 liter red wine (optional)

8 fluid ounces soy sauce, wheat free

1 bag plain rice cakes (salted OK)

8 ounce can oil-roasted peanuts

3.5 ounce package rice crackers

3 ounce can water-packed tuna fish

1 pound dry brown rice

1 pound granulated sugar

8 ounces pumpkin seeds

2 14.5 fluid ounce cans chicken broth

1 pound rice or corn rotini or small shell pasta

2 ounces baked potato chips

14.5 ounce can creamed yellow corn

Italian seasoning

Onion powder

Garlic powder

Dried basil

1 loaf wheat-free bread, such as Glutino brand

Produce

1 cup cauliflower florets

3 cups broccoli florets

1 head lettuce

1 pound mixed salad greens

3 tomatoes

1 pound baby carrots

2 pints cherry or grape tomatoes

2 cucumbers

5 pounds potatoes

1 large sweet potato

1 pound carrots

4 green bell peppers

2 red bell peppers

1 small eggplant

1 pound fresh baby spinach

10 ounce package fresh mushrooms

1 bunch bananas

4 tangerines

2 small oranges

2 pints fresh blueberries

1 pint fresh strawberries

Dairy Case

½ gallon lactose-free skim milk, such as Lactaid

4 ounce tub margarine

8 ounce carton sour cream

1 pound lactose-free cottage cheese, such as Lactaid

8 ounce package low-fat mozzarella cheese sticks

1 dozen eggs

2 ounces parmesan cheese

8 fluid ounce bottle orange juice

8 ounce package corn tortillas

6 ounce package low-fat cheese

Meat/Fish/Poultry

6 ounces deli sliced turkey

2 ounces deli sliced lean roast beef

6 ounces fresh salmon

15 ounces boneless, skinless chicken

6 ounces pork loin

1 pound raw, 90% lean ground beef

3 ounces steak

12 ounces lean ground turkey

1 pound cooked shrimp

Frozen

1 pint strawberry sorbet with allowed ingredients, such as Ciao Bella

12 ounce bag frozen, mixed allowed vegetables

Step 8: Vary Your Diet with Choices from the Allowed Food Lists

For the two-week duration of the elimination phase, eat only foods specifically named on the following lists as *allowed* foods. If a food does not appear on an allowed foods list, do not eat it. Later, you will be able to experiment with any food you desire. For the first two weeks, eat only allowed foods, simply prepared. In other words, be aware of sauces and other additions to your food. Make sure they, too, are allowed.

For prepared or processed foods on the lists, please read labels to make sure all ingredients are allowed. For example, turkey is an allowed food. You should either roast the turkey yourself (from a bird packaged with no problem ingredients) or ask to check the label on the processed turkey at the deli. For a detailed list of allowed food ingredients, please see the Appendix.

Limit yourself to the serving sizes suggested for all fruits, sweets and other foods in **bold-face type**. Choose only one of these foods per meal. For all other foods, portion sizes are suggestions only.

Allowed Grains/Starches

All of the foods on this list are allowed because they are either known to be, or likely to be, low in *fructans* (the goal is less than .5 grams of fructans per serving).[34] Note that only wheat-free grains and starches are allowed. Serving sizes are suggestions.

Allowed Foods	Serving Size
Cheerios	½ cup
Corn flakes	½ cup
Corn or rice pasta, cooked	½ cup
Corn tortillas	6 inch
Crackers: rice, corn or rye	14 small
Grits, uncooked	2 tablespoons
Kasha (buckwheat groats), cooked	½ cup
Oatmeal, cooked	½ cup
Popcorn, low-fat	2 cups
Potato, boiled or baked	½ cup or ½ medium
Potato chips	1 ounce
Puffed rice	1 ounce
Pumpkin, cooked	1 ½ cups
Rice or popcorn cakes, plain (salted OK)	3 large
Rice, brown or white, cooked	1/3 cup
Rutabaga, cooked	¾ cup
Rye crispbread, wheat-free	2 pieces
Soba noodles (buckwheat), cooked	½ cup
Squash, winter, cooked	1 cup
Tortilla chips	1 ounce
Sweet potato, baked	½ cup
Turnips, cooked	1/3 cup

Label Reading Tips for Grains/Starches

Please read labels carefully and avoid the following:

- Wheat as a major ingredient, including wheat flour, white flour, enriched flour and whole wheat flour (check cereals, breads, crackers, pastas, cookies, cake, pastries, muffins, bagels, pizza, sauces, gravies)

- Kamut and spelt, which are particular varieties of wheat (check cereals, breads, crackers, pastas, cookies, cake, pastries, muffins, bagels, pizza, sauces, gravies)

- Wheat berries or sprouted wheat (check breads)

- Inulin (check baked goods)

- Fructo-oligosaccharides/FOS (check low-fat cookies, granola or energy bars, cold/hot cereals)

- Fructose, crystalline fructose, high-fructose corn syrup (check baked goods, granola or energy bars, cold/hot cereals)

- Sorbitol, mannitol, isomalt, xylitol, maltitol, lactitol, polydextrose or hydrogenated starch hydrolysates (check energy and snack bars)

- Molasses (check baked goods)

These ingredients and descriptions are allowed:

- Wheat-derived minor ingredients such as wheat starch, maltodextrin and dextrose

- Gluten-free foods. Gluten-free claims on food labels may help you quickly identify wheat-free foods (although, as you know, gluten is not the part of wheat that you are avoiding). You should still read the label to check for the presence of other problem ingredients.

- Foods "produced in a facility that also makes products containing wheat." A trace of wheat in a product is not enough to cause problems with this diet.

⅏ *Allowed Fruits*

Fruits are the most limited food group on this elimination diet. You may be eating less fruit than usual. You can make up for this nutritionally by eating more vegetables, since fruits and vegetables provide many of the same nutrients.

Fruits with *more fructose than glucose* are not allowed on the basic diet. Fruits with a large quantity of *polyols* are not allowed on the basic diet. Fruits containing *fructans* are not allowed on the basic diet. All of the foods on this list are allowed because the fructose and glucose in the fruit are balanced (less than .5 grams excess/100 grams of food), the total fructose per serving is not too high and they are low in polyols and fructans.[35] [36] [37]

A note about bananas: as they ripen, the starches (polysaccharides) in the banana are converted to sugars.[38] The sugars are balanced, so ripe bananas in a limited portion are allowed on the basic diet. Clients often report that bananas cause constipation. Ripe bananas are likely to be better tolerated.

The serving size is critical for this food group. Allowed serving sizes are in bold-face type. If the total fructose load of the meal is too high, even if balanced with glucose, symptoms may occur.

Allowed Foods	Serving Size
Banana, ripe	**½ medium or large**
Blackberries	**½ cup**
Blueberries	**¾ cup**
Cranberries, raw	**1 cup**
Grapefruit juice	**1/3 cup**
Grapefruit	**½ large**
Lemon juice	**1/3 cup**
Lime juice	**1/3 cup**
Orange juice	**1/3 cup**
Orange	**1 small**

Raspberries	**1 cup**
Rhubarb	**½ cup**
Strawberries	**1 cup**
Tangelo	**1 medium**

Label Reading Tips for Fruits

Please read labels carefully and avoid the following:

- Fructose, crystalline fructose or high-fructose corn syrup (check fruit drinks or cocktails, fruit jam or jelly, fruit-flavored candy, sauces such as ketchup, plum sauce or chutney)

- Canned fruit packed in juice, not even allowed fruits

- Fruit-juice concentrate (check energy or snack bars, fruit drinks or cocktails, fruit spreads, fruit gummies, frozen fruit bars, cookies, sweets of any kind with "healthy" or "naturally sweetened" label claims

- Coconut milk or cream (check Indian and Thai foods)

- Fruit-juice based alcoholic drinks such as tequila sunrise, sea breeze, piña colada, mai tai, or daiquiri

⁄⁄ *Allowed Vegetables*

Vegetables containing large amounts of galactans or short-chain fructans are not allowed on your basic diet. A few vegetables have fructose in excess of glucose (more than 5 grams of fructose in excess of glucose per 100 grams). The following vegetables are allowed, because they contain only small amounts of galactans or short-chain fructans.

Serving sizes are suggestions.

Allowed Foods	Serving Size
Bamboo shoots	½ cup
Bean sprouts	1 cup
Bell pepper	1 medium
Beets	½ cup
Broccoli or broccoflower	1 cup florets or spears
Carrots	1 or ½ cup baby
Cauliflower	1 cup florets
Celery	4 medium stalks
Cherry tomatoes	8 or about 1 cup
Corn	½ cup
Cucumber	1 cup
Eggplant	1 cup
Kale, cooked	1 cup pieces
Lettuce	2 cups shredded
Mushrooms	1 cup whole
Peas, green	¼ cup
Radishes	10 small
Spinach, cooked	½ cup
Spinach, raw	2 cups
Tomato or tomatillo	1 medium or ½ cup
Water chestnuts	¾ cup
Pickle, dill or sour	1 large

Cooking Tip:

It is OK to cook with whole or large pieces of onion and garlic, which can be removed before consuming, even though the flesh of onion and garlic are not allowed. Onion and garlic powder can be used.

Label Reading Tips for Vegetables

Please read labels carefully and avoid the following:

- Tomato paste (check sauces, condiments, pizzas)
- Fructose, crystalline fructose or high-fructose corn syrup (check sauces, condiments, deli-prepared salads)

ℳ *Allowed Fats*

Nuts, seeds and olives are included in this group, because their primary contribution to the diet is fat. Oils from plant foods do not have any FODMAPS in them.

Milk-based fats usually contain *lactose*. Small serving sizes (bold-face type), with 2 grams or less of lactose per serving, are allowed on the basic diet. Serving sizes for other fats are suggestions.

Allowed Foods	**Serving Size**
Nuts, any type	½ ounce or 2 tablespoons
Oil, any type	1 teaspoon
Olives	9 large
Peanut butter	1 ½ tablespoons
Seeds, sesame or sunflower	1 tablespoon
Butter	1 teaspoon
Margarine	1 teaspoon
Mayonnaise, light	1 tablespoon
Mayonnaise, regular	2 teaspoons
Tartar sauce	1 tablespoon
Non-dairy topping	½ cup
Half-and-half	**2 tablespoons**
Sour cream	**1 ½ tablespoons**
Sour cream, low-fat	**1 ½ tablespoons**
Whipped cream	**4 tablespoons**
Cream cheese	**1 tablespoon**

Label Reading Tips for Fats

Please read labels carefully and avoid the following:

- ⃕ Inulin (check spreads, dressings, sauces, non-dairy toppings, low-fat sour cream and cream cheese)

- Fructose, crystalline fructose, or high-fructose corn syrup (check peanut butter, mayonnaise, non-dairy toppings)
- Fructo-oligosaccharides/FOS (check non-dairy toppings)

⅏ *Allowed Meats/Milk*

Protein is the major dietary contribution of foods in this group, including meat, fish, poultry, milk and milk products. If beans and lentils were a part of the basic diet, they would appear in this group as well. However, note there are no beans, dried peas or lentils on the allowed list for the basic diet, because they contain large amounts of galactans.

Some dairy products contain large amounts of lactose and are not allowed on the basic diet. lactose-free milk and milk products have been specially treated before packaging and are 100% lactose-free;[39] they are encouraged on the basic diet as excellent sources of protein, calcium and other nutrients. Dairy foods allowed on the basic diet contain 2 grams of lactose or less per serving. Limit serving sizes if food is shown in bold-face type.

Meat, fish and poultry without added ingredients do not contain FODMAPS. Serving sizes for those items are suggestions.

Allowed Foods	Serving Size
Almond milk	1 cup
Beef, lean	1 ½ ounces
Cheese, sharp cheddar or lactose-free	1 ounce
Cheese, low-fat sharp cheddar or lactose-free	2 ounces
Cheese, other	**1 ounce**
Cheese, shredded	**1/3 cup**
Cheese, cottage, lactose-free	1/2 cup
Cheese, ricotta, part-skim	**1/3 cup**
Chicken	2 ½ ounces
Clams	½ cup
Cod	3 ounces
Crab	3 ounces
Duck breast	3 ounces
Egg substitute	½ cup
Egg whites	4
Egg, whole	1

Fish	3 ounces
Halibut	3 ounces
Lamb, lean cuts	2 ounces
Milk, Lactose-free, skim or low-fat	1 cup
Pheasant	3 ounces
Pork, lean cuts	2 ounces
Salmon	3 ounces
Shrimp	3 ounces
Tilapia	3 ounces
Tuna	3 ounces or ½ cup
Turkey	3 ounces
Venison	3 ounces

Label Reading Tips for Meats/Milk

Please read labels carefully and avoid the following:

- Beans including baked beans, refried beans, kidney, pinto, black, edamame, lima, butter, navy, or garbanzo or any other dried beans, chick peas, black-eyed peas or any other dried peas (check soups, dips such as hummus, frozen meals, salads)

- Soy beans or soy products such as tofu, soy milk, tempeh (check vegetarian convenience foods, beverages)

- Lentils, including brown, yellow and red lentils (check soups, dal)

- Milk (unless it is pre-treated with lactase), nonfat dry milk powder, buttermilk or buttermilk solids

- Whey protein concentrate

- Yogurt or yogurt solids

These ingredients and descriptions are allowed:

- Foods "processed in a facility that also makes products containing milk"

- Whey protein isolate

⁂ *Allowed Extras*

Even allowed sweets must be limited in quantity on the basic diet, with a suggested maximum of 40 grams of total sugar per serving.[40] Some sweets contain *polyols* and are not allowed on the basic diet. Some sweets contain *excess fructose* and are not allowed on the basic diet. Sweets made with wheat flour, spelt or kamut contain *fructans* and are not allowed on the basic diet. The following foods are allowed in the quantities indicated:

Allowed Foods	Serving Size
Bakery items made with allowed ingredients	**1 ounce**
Candy made with allowed ingredients	**1 ounce**
Coffee, black, brewed	8 fluid ounces
Confectioners' sugar	**1 ½ tablespoons**
Granulated sugar	**1 ½ tablespoon**
Ice cream, lactose-free	**½ cup**
Jam or jelly	**1 ½ tablespoon**
Maple syrup, real	**1 ½ tablespoon**
Rice milk	1 cup
Sucrose-sweetened soft drink	**12 fluid ounces**
Sorbet with allowed ingredients	**½ cup**
Tea, black or green, brewed	8 fluid ounces
Wine, red or white	**4 fluid ounces**

Label Reading Tips for Extras

Please read labels carefully and avoid the following:

- ⸢ Honey

- Fructose, crystalline fructose or high-fructose corn syrup (check soft drinks/soda pop and other beverages, drink mixes, pancake syrup)

- Molasses or brown sugar (check gums, candies, beverages, energy or snack bars, cookies)

- Spelt, kamut or wheat flour in any form (check cakes, cookies, muffins, pastries)

- Beer, rosé wine, sweet alcoholic drinks such as margaritas, piña coladas, sweet martinis, sours and tropicals

- Ice cream, non-lactase treated

- Sorbitol, polydextrose, mannitol, isomalt, xylitol, maltitol, lactitol or hydrogenated starch hydrolysates (check liquid medications, flavored seltzer water and other beverages, gum, candy, nutrition and supplement bars)

- Inulin (check snack or energy bars, frozen desserts)

- Fructo-oligosaccharides/FOS (check low-fat cookies, granola bars, energy bars)

- Polydextrose (check frozen desserts)

These ingredients and descriptions are allowed:

- Table sugar, granulated sugar, cane sugar, dehydrated sugar cane juice, beet sugar, raw sugar, confectioners' sugar, sucrose

- Unsweetened spirits such as gin, vodka, whiskey

- Splenda, aspartame and saccharine

- Vinegar

- Wheat-free soy sauce

◢ *Beyond the Allowed Food Lists*

There are thousands of foods in the world that do not appear on the "allowed" food lists in this book. Some of them are specifically "not allowed" until the challenge phase of the diet. What about the many foods, beverages and ingredients that are not mentioned at all? They are not mentioned because I was unable to find published material about their nutrient composition or biochemical structure. Therefore, I couldn't definitively say whether they were allowed or not allowed.

Happily, this has the effect of keeping the FODMAPS elimination diet rather simple. It certainly doesn't mean that foods not mentioned in the book are off limits for you. Not at all; just avoid them during the elimination and challenge phases of the FODMAPS Elimination Diet. After the challenge phase of the diet is over, feel free to resume other foods that you tolerated in the past. You will find out soon enough if they cause your IBS symptoms to return.

Step 9: Rate Your Symptoms

During both the first and second week on the basic elimination diet, rate your symptoms on a symptom rating worksheet (see Appendix). Although this may seem somewhat tedious at times, it is very important.

Step 10: Assess Your Response to the Elimination Phase

If you are working with a dietitian, this is the time to meet again, approximately three weeks after your initial appointment.

If the FODMAPS Elimination Diet has done its job, you may be feeling so much better by now that you don't need any worksheets or numbers to tell you that. To confirm your impression, you can use your symptom worksheets to help you determine what to do next. If your results have been less dramatic, the worksheets will be especially helpful. At this point, you should have three weekly worksheets: one filled out before you started the elimination phase (your baseline), and one each for the first two weeks on the diet.

Let us recap how you will know whether the diet is working. Review the records and compare the symptoms you were experiencing at the baseline (before the diet) to the symptoms you experienced during weeks one and two of the diet. If the elimination is working, there should be a noticeable drop in the number and type of symptoms you experience; the numbers should have declined. The extent to which you benefit from the diet is ultimately your decision, using these numbers as a guide. You are the one who decides whether FODMAPS carbohydrates are the source of your IBS symptoms. You will come to one of two conclusions:

1. Your Symptoms Have Improved Markedly

If you decide that your symptoms have improved markedly, you should continue on to Chapter 5, which describes the challenge phase of the FODMAPS Elimination Diet.

2. Your Symptoms Have Not Improved or Have Only Improved a Little

If you follow this FODMAPS Elimination Diet faithfully and carefully for several weeks and you are still no better, it might be helpful to write down everything you eat and drink for a few days. Ask someone else to review the diet record with you and compare it to the allowed food lists, looking for unintentional sources of FODMAPS in the diet.

Have you been making exceptions for any reason? Unfortunately, exceptions will ruin your experiment. During the elimination phase you should not make any exceptions at all. If you find your diet wasn't as FODMAPS free as you had hoped, you may wish to continue the elimination phase for another week or two.

You may be aware of other possible factors that held back potential improvement in your symptoms, such as a particularly stressful week or a viral illness. If that is the case, continue the elimination phase for another two weeks and reassess.

If your diet has, indeed, been FODMAPS free for two weeks, and there are no other special circumstances to explain two weeks of continued symptoms, there is probably little to be gained by continuing. At this point, you should talk to your dietitian or doctor about other options.

Chapter 5
FODMAPS Carbohydrate Challenge

Step 11: Plan the FODMAPS Challenges

IF YOU HAVE seen a significant improvement in your symptoms during the elimination phase, you can move on to the challenge phase of the diet whenever you are ready. There is no big rush. If you are feeling well for the first time in years, go ahead and enjoy it for a while. The basic diet is healthy and nutritious.

It will take approximately six weeks to work your way through the challenge phase of the diet. After that, the process of experimenting with new foods can be ongoing.

When you are ready, choose a FODMAPS group to challenge. Do the one that is the most important to you first. Leave the foods you can easily do without for last. If you are expecting severe IBS symptoms to result from a challenge, be sure to plan it for a time when you can afford to deal with the symptoms for the next 24 hours.

You will probably be more sensitive to some FODMAPS than to others. That is the reason to do each challenge one at a time for a week, monitoring symptoms as you go along.

If you challenge more than one group at a time, you will not learn nearly as much. For example, if you challenge yourself by eating a pizza, you will not know whether your bloating and constipation the next morning resulted from eating the wheat in the crust, the lactose in the cheese or the tomato paste in the pizza sauce.

Since you will only be challenging with one type of FOD-MAPS carbohydrate at a time, you will have to eat quite a bit of it to get the total carbohydrate load you may have had from the combination of FODMAPS you were eating before.

If you already know that you don't tolerate a particular class of FODMAPS from years of hard-won personal experience, there is no need to put yourself through a challenge. For example, if you've known for years that you malabsorb lactose, and you get gas and diarrhea every time you consume it, you can skip the lactose challenge.

%%% Lactose Challenge

Dates of Lactose Challenge: _____
Foods to include during your lactose challenge:
> Cheese, larger servings
> Frozen yogurt, sweetened with sugar* only (no inulin or polydextrose)
> Ice cream, sweetened with sugar* only (no inulin or polydextrose)
> Milk, unflavored, all types
> Yogurt, cow's milk, sweetened with sugar* only (no inulin, high-fructose corn syrup or polydextrose)

*Sugars allowed include cane sugar, beet sugar, granulated sugar, confectioner's sugar, organic cane sugar, evaporated cane juice.

⁂ Fructose Challenge

Dates of Fructose Challenge: _____

Foods and ingredients to include during your fructose challenge:

Barbecue sauce

Carbonated non-diet soft drink

Catsup

Coconut milk or cream

Crystalline fructose

Dried fruit bars or leathers

Dried fruit, any type but raisins

Figs

Fructose

Fruit "drink" or punch

Fruit juice, any type but apple

Fruit spreads

Fruits on allowed list, larger servings

Granola or snack bars

High-fructose corn syrup

Honey

Ice tea made from mix or pre-made

Jam or jelly, commercially made

Lemonade made from mix or pre-made

Mangos

Melon, any type but watermelon

Molasses

Pancake syrup

Papayas

Plum sauce

Rosé wine

Sherry

Sweet and sour sauce

Tomato paste

▨ Fructans Challenge

Dates of Fructans Challenge: _____

Foods and ingredients to include during your fructans challenge:

    Artichokes
    Asparagus
    Bagel
    Banana, greener
    Beer
    Breads made of wheat
    Breakfast cereal made of wheat
    Cake
    Chicory-based coffee substitute
    Cookies
    Crackers made of wheat
    English muffin
    Flour tortilla
    Fructo-oligosaccharides
    Garlic
    Green onion
    Inulin
    Leeks
    Onions
    Pastry
    Pineapples
    Pizza dough made of wheat
    Sandwich or sub rolls made of wheat
    Shallots
    Spaghetti or pasta made of wheat
    Summer squash
    Zucchini

‰ Polyols Challenge

Dates of Polyols Challenge: _____
Foods and ingredients to include during your polyols challenge:

> Apricots
> Hydrogenated starch hydrolysates
> Isomalt
> Lactitol
> Low-calorie or lite frozen desserts
> Low-calorie, sweetened carbonated water
> Maltitol
> Mannitol
> Nectarines
> Plums
> Polydextrose
> Sorbitol
> Sugarless candy
> Sugarless gum
> Xylitol

‰ Special Case Fruits Challenge 1

Dates of Special Case Fruits Challenge 1: _____
Fruits in this group are high in both fructose and sorbitol. Foods to include during your Special Case Fruits 1 challenge:

> Apple cider
> Apple juice
> Applesauce
> Apples, any variety
> Apricots

Fruit juice blends including apple
Juice from canned fruit
Peaches
Pears
Prunes
Prune juice
Sweet cherries

﹉ Special Case Fruits Challenge 2

Dates of Special Case Fruits Challenge 2: _____
Fruits in this group are high in both fructose and fructans. Foods to include during your Special Case Fruits 2 challenge:

Grapes
Raisins
Mangos
Watermelon

﹉ Galactans Challenge

Dates of Galactans Challenge: _____
In one sense, galactans challenge is not necessary; we know that galactans will be malabsorbed in all cases. However, when symptoms have improved, you may try re-introducing the following to determine your tolerance level:

Baked beans, canned without molasses or high-fructose corn syrup
Black-eyed peas
Brussels sprouts
Cabbage
Dried or canned beans, all kinds
Dried peas, all kinds
Green beans
Hummus

Lentils
Soy-based vegetarian convenience food
Soy milk
Tempeh
Textured vegetable protein (TVP)
Tofu
Veggie burgers
Yellow beans

Step 12: Execute the Cautious Challenge

On the first day of the first challenge, eat just one or two normal servings of a food you used to eat routinely from the challenge group. This is a cautious test, in case you are so sensitive to that type of carbohydrate that even a small amount will provoke severe symptoms. For example, one of my clients with severe IBS and GERD used to eat wheat products several times a day. After two weeks on the basic diet, she was feeling so much better that she was reluctant to even consider doing any of the challenges. A few weekends later, however, she was on a camping trip. Rolls were on the menu, and there wasn't much other food available. It seemed like as good a time as any to challenge herself with carbohydrates from the fructans group. She decided to eat two rolls. On the way home the next morning, she also had a biscuit. This was enough to make her feel ill all week. When I saw her on Thursday, she was just starting to get over her unplanned fructans challenge.

Step 13: Execute the Big Challenge

If you haven't learned what you need to know after a cautious trial of the challenge group, give yourself a bigger challenge. Do not be tentative about it. You are *trying* to provoke symptoms. Eat the largest portions from the test group that might be typical for you. For example, if you are testing fructans, go ahead and eat a large bagel for breakfast along with a large greenish banana. Have pizza (no cheese yet) with onions and artichoke hearts on it for lunch. For dinner, how about a nice big plate of pasta with several cloves of baked garlic and sautéed zucchini on the side?

In this example, you could continue with the fructans challenge for several days to a week, but you can stop sooner if you are clearly experiencing painful or uncomfortable symptoms.

There is nothing to be gained by forcing yourself to eat FODMAPS foods beyond your usual portions. Overstuffing your stomach will not aid clarity here. The best way to assure a high intake of the test FODMAPS is to select multiple items from the test list at the same meal, all day long.

The galactans group is an exception. Do not consume dried peas, beans or lentils multiple times a day for the challenge. There is no need to do this because you are guaranteed to malabsorb galactans. Use smaller, more cautious amounts of high-galactans foods to explore how much of them you can tolerate without provoking symptoms. Some people find that their tolerance for galactans does improve over time with continued exposure to small and then gradually larger portions of food.

Step 14: Cycle Through All the Challenges

After each challenge, I recommend returning to the elimination phase basic diet for a few days. In other words, stop eating the FODMAPS that you just used for the challenge. This is especially important if you experience significant symptoms from one of the challenges.

When you are ready, select and carry out the next challenge. Do just one challenge at a time. Don't add challenges on top of each other at this time.

Step 15: Assess the Challenge Results

Challenge Causes No Symptoms

You may find that you have no increase in symptoms from some of the challenges. For example, if your body produces plenty of the enzyme lactase, you won't have trouble digesting lactose (milk sugar). If you challenge yourself with several generous helpings of regular milk products and experience no increase in gas, bloating, abdominal pain or diarrhea, you are free to enjoy milk products any time with no restrictions.

If the challenge group does not provoke symptoms, that is excellent news. However, you should continue to leave them out of your basic diet when you challenge with the next group. I do not recommend adding challenges on top of each other until after you have worked your way through the individual FODMAPS groups one-by-one.

Consider returning to the basic diet for a week before trying the next challenge, if you have significantly provoked your IBS symptoms.

Challenge Causes Severe Symptoms

There may be some FODMAPS foods that you choose to permanently drop from your diet. For example, I doubt that the client described earlier (who ate rolls and biscuits on the camping trip) will be eating wheat again any time soon. Now that she knows how sensitive she is to wheat, she will be equally cautious with all of the other foods in the fructans challenge group.

If you do have uncomfortable symptoms when challenging yourself, you will have learned something very important for your troubles. Discomfort=knowledge=power! The results are subjective. You decide if these are symptoms you can live with or not. Your symptom rating worksheets will be helpful to you as you decide how to proceed.

Challenge Causes Moderate Symptoms

There may be times when you are willing to risk a fair amount of discomfort in order to enjoy something really special, such as a big slice of Grandma's apple pie or a pizza once in a while. That's perfectly OK. There are some strategies you can use to make your symptoms more tolerable.

Planning ahead is the best strategy to use for eating events you know about in advance. If you know that lactose is a problem carbohydrate for you, and that the family is planning to go out for ice cream later in the day, you may choose to limit the amount of lactose and/or other FODMAPS that you consume at breakfast and lunch. Up to a point, you may be able to compensate for consuming troublesome FODMAPS after the fact. For example, if you are sensitive to fructans, you probably will try to limit the amount of wheat in your diet. Perhaps a given day got off to a bad start because the only food served at the breakfast meeting you attended was bagels. If you choose carefully for the rest of the day, avoiding most other FODMAPS, you may get away with it.

Chapter 6
Another Approach

THERE MAY BE times when it is appropriate to take the opposite approach to the elimination diet. As most of this book describes, I usually recommend eliminating all the FODMAPS at the beginning, then adding them back one by one to see what happens. Another approach would be to *remove* the FODMAPS one by one, keeping the rest of the usual diet intact.

The reason I usually prefer the first approach is that my clients, understandably, want to feel better immediately, if not sooner. They want to know within a week or two whether the FODMAPS Elimination Diet holds the answers for them.

However, removing FODMAPS one group at a time might be a better choice if you already have a lot of other dietary limitations or are not very flexible in your food preferences.

How would you know where to start? The following quiz will help you decide where to focus your efforts by figuring out which type of FODMAPS are most prominent in your diet. This quiz is not a scientifically validated screening tool; it is based on common sense. The foods you eat most often have a bigger influence on your health than the ones you eat once in a while. Also, you may be blind to your trigger foods because you were always told they were safe foods for IBS, such as white bread and pasta. You may be deliberately eating some FOD-MAPS-containing foods, such as apples and pears, for their well-known health benefits, without realizing they are causing you distress in other ways. Remember, "one man's meat is another man's poison"; you must discover which types of carbohydrates are right for you.

Quiz—Food Frequency Questionnaire

For each of the following foods, write down the number of serving or units **per week** you eat of that food in the space provided. *Do your best to add up your usual intake for an entire typical seven-day week.* If you have difficulty with these calculations, read the examples carefully and see if one of them can help you.

The serving size for many foods is described in terms of cups or tablespoons; for example, cottage cheese, ½ cup. You probably don't usually measure your cottage cheese before you eat it! Before you complete this questionnaire, get out some measuring cups and measuring spoons and remind yourself what ½ cup, 1 cup, 1 tablespoon and 1 teaspoon of food look like. Remember, the amount of food in the measuring cups and spoons should be level with the top, not "heaping." Measure some foods into your usual plates, bowls and cups. Picturing those quantities should make completing this questionnaire easier.

You can usually find out the weight of the foods you eat by checking the food label. One way to do this is to compare the weight of the whole package to the amount you eat in a week. Another way is to check the Nutrition Facts panel on the packaging. At the top of the panel you will usually find the serving size and weight in grams. If you are actually eating more than the listed serving size, be sure to take that into account. Thirty grams is roughly equal to 1 ounce.

Example 1: You eat pizza every Friday night. You eat 4 slices of pizza at that meal. The unit indicated for pizza is ½ slice. You would write "8" in the space provided.

Example 2: You eat 3 sandwiches per week on wraps. There are 8 wraps in a 16-ounce package. Therefore, each wrap weighs 2 ounces and is equal to 2 servings. You would write "6" in the space provided.

Example 3: You eat 4 cups of small crackers per week. The Nutrition Facts panel tells you the serving size is ½ cup (30 grams). Thirty grams is approximately one ounce. You are eating 8 times that amount, so you would write "8" in the space provided.

Example 4: You eat one very large cookie a week from the canteen at work. At your request, the cafeteria worker checks the frozen dough package for you and tells you the cookie weighs 3 ounces. You would write "3" in the space provided.

Note, there may be certain foods you eat only in season; write "0" for the number of servings of out-of-season foods, since you are not currently eating them.

Lactose Group

Cottage or ricotta cheese, ½ cup   _____
Cow's milk (not Lactaid), 8 fluid ounces   _____
Goat's milk, 8 fluid ounces   _____
Hot chocolate, 8 fluid ounces   _____
Ice cream, ½ cup   _____
Yogurt, any commercial variety, 6-8 ounces   _____
Yogurt, frozen, ½ cup   _____
Total servings lactose foods per week: _____

Fructose Group

Carbonated, non-diet soft drink,12 fluid ounces	_____
Catsup, 2 Tablespoon	_____
Coconut milk or cream, ¼ cup	_____
Dried fruit bars or fruit leathers, 1 whole	_____
Dried fruit, other than raisins, 2 tablespoons	_____
Fruit "drink" or punch, 8 fluid ounces	_____
Fruit juice, any type but apple or prune, 1/3 cup	_____
Granola or snack bars, 1 whole	_____
Honey, 1 ½ tablespoons	_____
Iced tea or lemonade, pre-made, 8 fluid ounces	_____
Jam/jelly, commercially made, 1 ½ tablespoons	_____
Melon, other than watermelon, ½ cup	_____
Pancake syrup (not real maple), 1 ½ tablespoons	_____
Papaya, ½ cup	_____
Sherry or port wine, 4 fluid ounces	_____
Sweet and sour/plum/BBQ sauce, 1 ½ tablespoons	_____
Tomato paste, 1 ½ Tablespoon	_____
Total servings of fructose foods per week:	_____

Fructans Group

Artichokes, ½ cup	_____
Asparagus, ½ cup	_____
Beer, 12 fluid ounces	_____
Cake, 1 piece	_____
Cookies, 1 ounce	_____
Pastry, 1 piece	_____
Chicory-based coffee substitute, 8 fluid ounces	_____
Garlic, 1 clove	_____
Leeks, ½ cup	_____
Onions, ½ cup	_____
Breakfast cereal made of wheat, ½ cup	_____
Bread, white or whole wheat, 1 ounce	_____
Pizza, ½ slice	_____
Sandwich or sub rolls, 3" length	_____
English muffin, ½	_____
Bagel, 1 ounce or ¼ bagel	_____
Flour tortilla or roll-up, 1 ounce	_____

Crackers made of wheat, 1 ounce _____
Spaghetti or pasta, ½ cup cooked _____
Total servings of fructans foods per week: _____

Polyols Group

Apricots, 2 small _____
Liquid medications, 1 dose—do not discontinue
without guidance from the prescribing physician _____
Sweetened seltzer water, 8 fluid ounces _____
Nectarines, 1 medium _____
Plums, 2 small _____
Sugarless candy, 1 ounce _____
Sugarless gum, 1 stick or piece _____
Low-cal or lite frozen desserts, ½ cup or 1 piece _____
Total servings polyols foods per week: _____

Special Case Fruits Group 1:

(High in both fructose and sorbitol)
Apple, 1 medium _____
Applesauce, ½ cup _____
Apple cider, 1/3 cup _____
Apple juice, 1/3 cup _____
Cherries, sweet, ½ cup _____
Fruit juice blends including apple, 8 fluid ounces _____
Juice from canned fruit, 1/3 cup _____
Nectarines, 1 medium _____
Peaches, 1 medium _____
Pear, 1 medium _____
Prunes, 4 _____
Prune juice, 1/3 cup _____
Total servings special case fruits per week: _____

Special Case Fruits Group 2:

(High in both fructose and fructans)
Grapes, ½ cup _____
Mangos, ½ cup _____
Raisins, 2 tablespoons _____
Watermelon, ½ cup _____

Galactans Group

Baked beans, ½ cup   _____
Beans, green or yellow, ½ cup   _____
Dried peas/beans, cooked or canned, ½ cup   _____
Brussels sprouts, ½ cup   _____
Cabbage, ½ cup   _____
Health, energy or nutrition bars   _____
Hummus, ½ cup   _____
Lentils, ½ cup   _____
Soy milk, ½ cup   _____
Tempeh, ½ cup   _____
Textured vegetable protein, ½ cup   _____
Tofu, ½ cup   _____
Veggie burgers or other soy-based
vegetarian convenience foods   _____
Total servings of galactans foods per week: _____

Questionnaire Summary

Write in the total servings per week for each of the following food groups:

Lactose   _____
Fructos   _____
Fructans   _____
Polyols   _____
Special Case Fruits 1   _____
Special Case Fruits 2   _____
Galactans   _____

Applying Results of the Food Frequency Questionnaire

As you review your food frequency questionnaire summary, you may see a group that clearly emerges as the primary source of FODMAPS in your diet. That is the group you should elimi-nate first in this alternate approach to the FODMAPS Elimi-nation Diet. Before you start, however, please take a week to rate your symptoms using a symptom rating worksheet (see Appendix) to establish a baseline symptom profile. Rating your symptoms will be extremely helpful later for deciding whether elimination of a particular food group makes a difference for you.

Next, select one group of FODMAPS from the food frequency questionnaire to eliminate. For seven days, do not eat any of the foods listed in that section of the questionnaire (important exception—do not discontinue prescribed liquid medications without guidance from the prescribing physician). For example, if you are eliminating the Lactose Group, for one week do not eat or drink any regular (untreated) cottage cheese, milk, hot chocolate, yogurt, frozen yogurt or ice cream. Don't make any exceptions, just for this one week. Rate and record your symptoms during the week. If there is a noticeable reduction in your symptoms, compared to the baseline week, you may have discovered that you do not tolerate that type of FODMAPS carbohydrate well.

Return to your usual diet, including the tested group, for a few days. Do your symptoms return?

Work your way through each group, giving yourself a few days in between to return to your usual diet.

See the section entitled, "How to Use Your New Information," for advice on how to proceed after you have tested all the food groups.

Chapter 7
Understanding Carbohydrate Malabsorption

What are Carbohydrates?

ARBOHYDRATES ARE SUBSTANCES in food that consist of a single sugar molecule or multiples of them in various forms. They provide the body with energy.[41] [42] The other two energy-providing nutrients are protein and fat. Although protein and fat are important parts of the diet, it is the carbohydrates that seem to be of great importance in contributing to FODMAPS-sensitive IBS.

Many foods provide a combination of protein, carbohydrates and fats. Significant amounts of carbohydrates are found in sweets, sweetened beverages, cereals and grains, fruits, vegetables and milk products. Little or no carbohydrates are present in meat, fish, poultry, nuts, seeds, fats or oils.

Sugars are the most basic type of carbohydrate. *Monosaccharides* consist of just one sugar molecule, all by itself. Examples of monosaccharides include glucose (blood sugar), fructose (fruit sugar) and galactose. *Disaccharides* consist of two sugar molecules linked together. Examples include table sugar (sucrose), malt sugar (maltose) and milk sugar (lactose). *High-fructose corn syrup* consists of sugars as well. *Polyols*, or sugar alcohols, are considered sugars.[43] Examples of polyols are sorbitol, xylitol and mannitol.

Complex carbohydrates are also known as *oligosaccharides* and *polysaccharides*. Some examples of complex carbohydrates are starches and dietary fiber. *Starches* consist primarily of long, interlocking chains of glucose or fructose units. Examples of foods containing large amounts of starch are rice, wheat, corn and potatoes. Most starches can be digested and absorbed by the human body ("modified" starch is less digestible). *Dietary fiber* consists of non-digestible complex carbohydrates found in plants. Dietary fiber is poorly broken down by human digestive enzymes. Well-known sources of dietary fiber include whole grains, dried peas and beans, fruits and vegetables.

Digestion and Absorption of Carbohydrates

Digestion of carbohydrates begins in your mouth. Your teeth chew and grind the food, mixing it with saliva. Saliva contains enzymes that begin the process of breaking carbohydrates down.

Carbohydrates in your food are further broken down by enzymes in your small intestine. If they are fully digested, they are broken down to their basic units of glucose, fructose and galactose. These simple sugars then must pass through the lining of the small intestine into the blood stream, where they are carried off to serve as fuel for your body. Glucose, fructose and galactose are the *only* carbohydrates that are absorbed by the human body.

What Is Malabsorption?

If anything prevents carbohydrates from being broken down or passing through the lining of the small intestine, they cannot be absorbed, and *malabsorption* is said to occur. There are many possible causes of malabsorption, among them:

- Lack, or shortage, of the necessary digestive enzymes. This is a common cause of lactose (milk sugar) malabsorption in adults.

- Fast intestinal transit time; food is catapulted through your system without enough time for digestive enzymes to work.

- Total amount of sugar in the meal exceeds the capacity of the small intestine to digest and absorb it.

- Composition of the meal; fructose is absorbed more completely in the presence of glucose and less completely in the presence of sugar alcohols.

- Damage to the lining of the small intestine, for example, from food poisoning, a virus, untreated celiac disease or Crohn's disease.

- Short bowel syndrome; if any length of the small intestine has been surgically removed, malabsorption can occur.

- Some carbohydrates, the dietary fibers such as those found in wheat bran or beans, are never digested or absorbed in the small intestine. Humans do not have the digestive enzymes to break down these dietary fibers.

When carbohydrates are malabsorbed, they pass to the end of the small intestine and into the large intestine, where they can cause chaos for individuals with FODMAPS-sensitive IBS.

Osmosis

Normally, one of the main functions of your large intestine is to reabsorb water from your stool into your bloodstream, turning it from a liquid into more of a solid form, ready for excretion.

Some carbohydrates, when malabsorbed, interfere with this process. Instead, they may cause water to be pulled into the stool. This happens through the process of *osmosis.* Osmosis in this setting is the movement of water through semi-permeable cell membranes, attracted by a higher concentration of sugar inside the lumen of the large intestine. The resulting watery bowel movement is sometimes termed *osmotic diarrhea.*

The best way to picture osmosis is to think of what happens when you sprinkle sugar on a bowl of freshly cut strawberries. The sugar pulls the liquid out of the strawberries and pretty soon you have a large volume of strawberry juice in the bowl. You have witnessed osmosis. The sugar is *osmotically active*, in other words capable of pulling the juice (water) through the cell walls of the strawberries and into the bowl.

A common characteristic of FODMAPS is their high osmotic activity. If they are present in your stool in a high concentration, they are capable of pulling water from your body into the large intestine.[44]

Fermentation

Your large intestine is populated by millions of bacteria. That is normal. Bacteria need energy to survive, and they get it by consuming the simple sugars and complex carbohydrates that were not absorbed earlier in the digestive process. Although humans do not have the enzymes to digest dietary fiber, bacteria do.

Fermentation is the breakdown of carbohydrates by bacteria. Energy is produced to keep the bacteria alive. Waste products of fermentation are short-chain fatty acids, hydrogen gas, carbon dioxide gas and, in some individuals, methane gas. Some of these gasses are, in turn, consumed by bacteria in the colon, yielding acetate, methane, sulfates and hydrogen sulfide. Unused gasses are absorbed and excreted in the breath or excreted through the anus. [45]

Some carbohydrates are fermented more rapidly than others. FODMAPS are all rapidly fermentable.[46] They make it possible for bacteria to produce a lot of gas in a short amount of time, causing problems for some IBS sufferers.

On the flip side, it should be noted, the short-chain fatty acids produced by bacteria in your large intestine are thought to have some health benefits, and serve as the primary nutrient for the epithelial cells lining the colon.[47] Some FODMAPS are specifically added to foods to stimulate fermentation by so-called good bacteria and their production of short chain fatty acids.[48] These additives are sometimes termed *prebiotics*, and include inulin and fructo-oligosaccharides (FOS). These additives may increase symptoms due to fermentation in some individuals.[49] (The term *pre*biotic is distinct from the term *pro*biotic. Probiotics are the "good bacteria" that are sometime deliberately ingested for purported health benefits. Prebiotics are preferred carbohydrate foods for those good bacteria. Some supplements and foods contain both, to stimulate increased activity of the good bacteria.)

Hydrogen Breath Testing

A laboratory test called *hydrogen breath testing* is based on the fact that fermentation of malabsorbed carbohydrates results in bacterial production of excess hydrogen gas. The gas is absorbed into the bloodstream and excreted in the breath, where it can be measured.

Your physician can order hydrogen breath testing to check for fructose malabsorption. Fructose is only one of the FOD-MAPS. Why single it out? Why is it helpful to know whether you malabsorb fructose? Screening for fructose malabsorption turns out to be one of the best ways to identify people who are likely to be helped by the FODMAPS Elimination Diet. Not everyone with IBS malabsorbs fructose. Of those who do, however, studies suggest that up to 85 percent respond to a fructose-controlled diet with reduced symptoms.[50] [51]

It is not essential to be tested for fructose malabsorption, however. You can just as easily try the FODMAPS Elimination Diet for a couple of weeks and observe your symptoms. They should tell you a great deal about whether you have a problem absorbing fructose. If the situation is unclear, however, and you choose to pursue testing, it is available at many labs and medical centers. Because the testing procedure takes place over several hours, it is more likely to be offered at a hospital laboratory rather than at a satellite phlebotomy clinic.

To prepare for the test, you will be asked to fast for 12 hours before your appointment, and to refrain from smoking or brushing your teeth for two hours before the testing procedure begins. You should not have the test within two weeks of taking antibiotics.

Every laboratory has its own protocols for laboratory testing, but the following is a possible scenario. At the beginning of the test, your breath will be collected to establish a baseline. Then you will be given a solution of 25 grams of fructose dissolved in water. Your breath will be collected every 30 minutes over a three-hour period. The hydrogen in your breath will be measured. If there is a 20 parts per million difference between the baseline and any of the follow-up breath samples, your test is considered positive.[52] Some labs test for methane gas in your breath as well.

Breath testing for lactose malabsorption is also available, but it is rarely performed. It is easy enough to figure out whether you tolerate lactose by dropping milk and milk products from your diet for a couple of weeks. If your symptoms improve on a milk-free diet, and worsen again when you challenge yourself with milk, you will know that you probably malabsorb lactose to some degree.

Limitations of Breath Testing

In Australia and New Zealand, IBS patients are routinely screened for fructose malabsorption. At some medical centers there, patients who are positive for both IBS and fructose malabsorption are immediately referred for dietary counseling to reduce intake of fructose and other FODMAPS.

In the United States, hydrogen breath testing is done less often. One problem with hydrogen breath testing is that it is not specific for fructose malabsorption. There are other reasons why your test could be positive for hydrogen in your breath, including invasion of the small intestine by bacteria normally only present in the colon (this is called small intestine bacterial overgrowth, or SIBO).[53]

There are several additional reasons that the test could fail to give a positive result even if you do have fructose malabsorption. Diarrhea or active bowel disease can interfere with the outcome of the test. The dose of fructose given (usually 25 grams) may not be high enough to provoke symptoms in some individuals. In research settings, up to 50 grams of fructose may be given to measure fructose malabsorption.[54] [55] If an individual is a methane producer, and the lab does not analyze breath samples for methane, the test could fail to give a positive result.

Finally, studies have shown that not everyone who malabsorbs fructose experiences IBS symptoms. It is likely that an underlying susceptibility to IBS (such as visceral hypersensitivity or a motility disorder) has to also be present for symptoms to occur.[56]

Chapter 8
Understanding FODMAPS Carbohydrates

A S YOU LEARNED in Chapter 3, FODMAPS stands for Fermentable **O**ligo-, **D**i- and **M**ono-saccharides **A**nd **P**olyols. Specifically, some of the dietary carbohydrates described by the term, FODMAPS, are lactose, fructose, fructans, polyols and galactans. This chapter provides more details about each of these.

Lactose

Lactose is the primary sugar present in milk. It is a disaccharide of glucose and galactose. Lactose is broken down by the enzyme lactase in the small intestine. Many people don't produce enough lactase, and can't break lactose down to glucose and galactose so it can be absorbed. Lack of the enzyme lactase can be temporary. For example, when a lactose-malabsorbing individual with celiac disease or Crohn's disease achieves remission, sometimes his or her ability to produce lactase may return. That individual might then be able to consume lactose without symptoms.

Lactose insufficiency is very rarely seen in infants and young children. However, up to 90 percent of adults have some degree of lactose malabsorption, particularly those of African, Jewish, Native-American, Mexican and Asian descent.[57] In parts of the world (especially northern Europe) where the climate allows dairy cows to be raised, milk and milk products are a major part of the economy and cuisine. Interestingly, people descended from northern Europe tend to retain the ability to digest lactose into adulthood, at least to some degree.

Untreated milk, either plain or flavored, has 11–15 grams of lactose in a one-cup serving.[58] Fermented milk products such as yogurt and kefir have slightly less lactose because the bacteria in those products break down some of the lactose. Untreated milk, yogurt and kefir are not allowed on the basic diet.

Hard cheeses, which have the whey drained off during processing, contain little or no lactose, and are allowed on the basic diet. Sour cream and butter have only a trace of lactose.

Lactaid-brand milk and milk products have been pre-treated with the enzyme lactase. The enzyme breaks lactose down to its simple sugars, and the resulting products are 100 percent lactose free.[59] This brand is widely available in grocery stores in the United States and Canada. Other brands of lactose-free milk and milk products may be available in your area, as well.

Don't make the mistake of jumping to the conclusion that milk products don't have anything to do with your IBS, because you can sometimes consume milk without experiencing symptoms. As you now know, this may have as much to do with the fact that you may have eaten less of the other FODMAPS on those "good" days. Don't make any assumptions about milk products, and do eliminate untreated milk on the basic diet.

Fructose

Fructose is a simple sugar that is found in three main forms in the diet:[60]

- ⮞ *Free fructose* is found in honey, high-fructose corn syrup and in fruits.[61] [62] The ratio of fructose and glucose varies and is unique in each of these foods.

- ⮞ Fructose is bound together with glucose in the form *sucrose* (table sugar); sucrose contains an equal amount of fructose and glucose.

- ⮞ Fructose molecules are bound together in long, repeating chains, *fructans*, which are discussed separately.

When the amount of fructose is equal to the amount of glucose in a food, it is absorbed more completely.[63] That is why it is OK to eat small portions of certain fruits and table sugar on the FODMAPS basic diet. However, even though fructose and glucose are balanced in these allowed foods, if the amount consumed is too large, the total amount of fructose may still be enough to cause problems. Therefore, on the allowed food lists for the basic diet, you will find that the serving sizes for fruits and sweets of all kinds are limited.

Pure corn syrup does not contain fructose, although Karo "corn syrup" does.[64] The term "high-fructose corn syrup" is used to refer to products ranging from 45 percent to 90 percent fructose.[65] Since one cannot tell from the ingredients list on a food label which product was used, and whether fructose is in excess of glucose, on the FODMAPS basic diet I recommend avoiding them all.

Intake of fructose in the U.S. has risen significantly since 1970, when high-fructose corn syrup began to replace sucrose as the preferred sweetener in the food industry, from an estimated 8.8 percent of calories in the 1970s to 11.5 percent of calories by the 1990s.[66] Adolescents, ages 12 to 18, consume the most fructose. Non-Hispanic blacks are the racial/ethnic group with the highest fructose intake.[67]

Fructans

Fructans, a type of oligosaccharides, are chains of the sugar fructose. These chains vary in length, and it is the shorter chains that probably cause the most problems due to fermentation and osmotic activity.[68] However, longer-chain fructans, sometime called *inulins*,[69] are also capable of causing symptoms.[70]

Short-chain fructans are often referred to as *fructooligosaccharides* (FOS).[71] They are found in a number of fruits and vegetables, notably garlic, onions, zucchini, watermelon, bananas, peaches, pineapples and grapes.

Fructans are not digested and absorbed in the small intestine. Humans do not produce an enzyme capable of breaking the fructose-fructose bonds present in fructans.[72]

Some fruits contain large amounts of both fructose and fructans, including grapes, raisins and watermelon. During the challenge phase of the diet, these fruits are included in the "Special Case Fruits Challenge 2."

Inulin is added to some brands of yogurt for fiber and to promote the activity of so-called "good" bacteria in the gut. This may be a mixed blessing for FODMAPS-sensitive IBS sufferers. FOS may be added to some products for the same reason.

Wheat deserves special mention here, as it is the largest source of fructans in the American diet, supplying approximately 70 percent of the fructans consumed.[73] When wheat is the main ingredient in a product, as it is in bread, some cereals, pasta, crackers and baked goods, it is capable of causing IBS symptoms in sensitive individuals.

Wheat is such a staple for most Americans that they never suspect it could be causing their symptoms; this culprit is hiding in plain sight. In fact, clients may say, "How could the problem be wheat? I eat wheat every day, and some days I feel fine!" Eliminating fruits, vegetables, milk, and dried peas and beans (but not wheat) does help symptoms drop back to a more manageable level, because it reduces the total FODMAPS load. One is left with little diversity in the diet, and a lot of empty calories.

If you discover that wheat causes your IBS symptoms to worsen, you will have learned something very important. It probably will not mean that you must always avoid wheat; it means that you choose the amount and frequency of wheat very carefully, to keep IBS symptoms under control.

Polyols

Polyols are osmotically active and strong laxatives in large doses, even for people without IBS.[74] [75] This characteristic is often deliberately exploited and probably explains the reputation of prunes and apples for preventing simple constipation. *Sorbitol*, one type of polyol, occurs naturally in some fruits; in addition to prunes and apples, it is found in apricots, nectarines, peaches, plums, sweet cherries and pears. Chemically, polyols resemble both sugars and alcohols; that is why they are often called sugar alcohols.

Other polyols derived from corn, sugar cane or whey are used as additives to sweeten sugarless gum, candy and some low-carb meal replacement bars. The list of ingredients in such foods might include *xylitol, sorbitol, mannitol, maltitol, erythritol, isomalt, lactitol or hydrogenated lactitol or hydrogenated starch hydrolysates.*[76] Erythritol seems to be an exception to the rule; although it is a sugar alcohol, it is appears to be well absorbed by humans in the small intestine, and not fermentable by colonic bacteria.[77] Therefore, it is not a FODMAP.

Polydextrose, while not a sugar alcohol, is derived from sorbitol and has FODMAPS properties.[78][79]

Fructose is not as well absorbed by the human body in the presence of polyols. Individuals who malabsorb fructose may have an especially difficult time tolerating apples, peaches, plums, prunes, sweet cherries and pears, all of which are high in both free fructose and sorbitol. During the challenge phase of the diet, these particular fruits are included in "Special Case Fruits Challenge 1".

Some liquid medications are sweetened with polyols. If you take liquid medications on a regular basis, check with your pharmacist to find out what your medication is sweetened with, and whether the medication is available in another form. Never discontinue a prescribed liquid medication without the guidance of the prescribing physician.

Galactans

Galactans are another type of oligosaccharide, the "O" in the acronym, FODMAPS. Galactans are chains of the sugar galactose. The primary dietary sources of galactans are certain legumes, such as baked beans, kidney beans, chick peas, soy products and so on. Galactans are also present in green and yellow (wax) beans, cabbage and brussels sprouts.

Galactans, like fructans, are almost entirely malabsorbed in all people, because humans do not produce an enzyme capable of breaking the galactose-galactose bond.[80] Galactans in the large intestine are highly fermentable and osmotically active. They can be relied on to cause gas, and give beans their reputation as the "musical fruit."

Conclusion

THE METHOD DESCRIBED in this book may be the beginning of a lifelong journey for you. By using the knowledge you have earned completing the step-by-step FODMAPS Elimination Diet, it is my hope that you will be IBS-free at last. You will be able to truly enjoy eating nutritious food, and nagging, unbearable symptoms will no longer prevent you from reaching your goals. I hope that you will experience the emotional relief and peacefulness that comes from feeling healthy.

There will be many challenges ahead, such as figuring out the effects of overlapping, multiple groups of FODMAPS. I know you will be looking for advice on adapting recipes, eating out, limiting FODMAPS in a family situation and more. I have created a web log, *www.ibsfree.net*, to accompany this book, in which I address these and many other subjects. Please visit me there. I look forward to hearing from you.

Acknowledgements

T HIS BOOK WOULD not exist without the pioneering research and clinical experience of Susan J. Shepherd, Peter R. Gibson and Jacqueline S. Barrett at the Box Hill Hospital in Victoria, Australia. Their work has made a tremendous difference to many patients in their IBS clinic and beyond. I look forward to meeting them some day.

I would like to thank Susan Quimby, RD, LD, for her trust in me and for mentoring me in my practice at Nutrition Works, LLC, in Portland, Maine. The support, encouragement and advice of my Nutrition Works colleagues Kim Norbert, Judy Donnelly, Janet Steady and Sharon Smalley, is very important to me, as well.

My husband, Paul Catsos, has been a loving and enthusiastic supporter during the writing of this book. I would like to thank him for reading the manuscript and offering critical feedback at several different points in the process. My children have been patient with me and have contributed to many off-color, and hilarious, mealtime brainstorming sessions for diet and book titles.

Numerous readers provided invaluable comments and questions to make this a better book, including Christine Catsos, Suzanne Danehy, Alena Prusinowski, Charles and Antoinette Tarbell, Kim Norbert and Susan Quimby.

I would also like to thank Linda Fullerton Hersey for copy editing and proofreading the text, and for sharing her journalism and publishing expertise with me.

Appendix

Recipes

I NCLUDED HERE ARE just four recipes that are referred to in the week of sample menus for the basic diet. All of the recipes provided are allowed on the basic diet. It is assumed that in all cases you will read labels for any commercially prepared ingredients and make sure that you buy a version of the product that is allowed.

If you are a more adventurous cook and would like to explore and modify other recipes, there are many world cuisines to explore that do not rely on wheat to the degree that Americans and Europeans do. To name just a few, try Chinese, Japanese, Thai, Indian, Mexican or Greek recipes.

There are many excellent gluten-free cookbooks on the market, if you want to broaden your horizons. Gluten-free recipes are automatically wheat-free, so these recipes may be a good place to start. Of course, you will have to screen all of the ingredients in recipes, even gluten-free recipes, to make sure that only allowed ingredients are included.

Peanut Butter Cookies

Thanks to my friend Antoinette Tarbell for this easy and delicious recipe.

INGREDIENTS:

1 egg
1 cup peanut butter (natural or standard types both work)
1 cup granulated sugar

DIRECTIONS:

- Preheat oven to 350° F.

- Mix ingredients well.

- Form into 1-inch balls or drop by rounded teaspoons on to ungreased cookie sheet.

- Press with the back of a sugared fork to make a crisscross design on top of each cookie.

- Bake 10–12 minutes, until the cookies look dry on top.

- Let cookies cool on the cookie sheets before removing and storing in an air-tight container.

Makes 28 small cookies.

Shepherd's Pie

Comfort food.

INGREDIENTS:

1 pound (raw) 90% lean ground beef
3 cups frozen, mixed and allowed vegetables
½ teaspoon onion powder
1 teaspoon garlic powder
14.5 ounce can creamed yellow corn
4 medium (approximately 3" long) potatoes
2 teaspoons reduced-fat margarine or butter
¼ cup lactose-free milk
salt and pepper to taste

DIRECTIONS:

- Preheat oven to 350°.

- Brown crumbled ground beef in skillet. Drain off any fat that accumulates.

- Combine frozen vegetables with ground beef and warm through. Add onion and garlic powder.

- Peel and boil potatoes until tender. Drain. Mash together with reduced-fat margarine or butter. Season with salt and pepper, if desired.

- Spread the ground beef mixture across the bottom of a 4-quart casserole dish. Spoon the corn evenly across the ground beef. Add all of the mashed potatoes in a layer across the top. Use the back of a spoon to smooth the surface.

- Bake for 45 minutes, until top of potatoes are golden brown.

Makes 4 servings

Shrimp Pasta Primavera

INGREDIENTS:

8 ounces (dry) rice or corn rotini or shells
2 tablespoons olive oil
2 cups broccoli florets
1 large or 2 small red bell peppers, chopped
1 cup eggplant, sliced into ¼ inch pieces
¼ cup green peas
¼ teaspoon Italian seasoning
1 teaspoon onion powder
½ teaspoon garlic powder
1 pound cooked shrimp
1 pint grape or cherry tomatoes, halved
Salt and pepper to taste
1 ounce (1/4 cup) shredded parmesan cheese

DIRECTIONS:

- Cook and drain pasta according to package directions.
- Meanwhile, heat oil in large skillet on medium heat. Add all vegetables (except tomatoes), Italian seasoning, onion and garlic powder. Sauté, stirring occasionally, until vegetables are tender.
- Add cherry tomatoes and cooked shrimp. Heat until tomatoes and shrimp are warmed through.
- Add cooked pasta to the skillet and stir gently.
- Salt and pepper to taste, if desired.
- Sprinkle with parmesan cheese.

Makes 4 large servings

Meatball Soup

This soup is a variation on Italian Wedding Soup.

INGREDIENTS:

12 ounces 90% lean ground beef or turkey
1 egg
2 tablespoons quick oats
1 tablespoon grated parmesan cheese
½ teaspoon dried basil
½ teaspoon onion powder
2 cans (each 14.5 fluid ounces) chicken broth
2 carrots
4 cups baby spinach leaves
2 cups cooked rice or corn rotini or small shells

DIRECTIONS:

- Combine ground beef, egg, oats, parmesan cheese, basil and onion powder. Form into 1" balls.

- Brown meatballs in non-stick skillet. Drain fat.

- In large saucepan, bring chicken broth to a boil.

- Stir in carrots, meatballs, cooked rice or pasta and meatballs.

- Simmer gently until spinach is tender.

Makes 4 servings

Summary of Label Reading Tips

Avoid foods that do not appear on the "allowed" lists in Chapter 4, Step 8. This section summarizes some common food additives that you may encounter on food labels as well as some tricky synonyms for wheat. You can tear out or copy this page and bring it to the grocery store with you.

Allowed:

Aspartame

Beet sugar

Cane sugar

Confectioner's sugar

Dehydrated sugar cane juice

Dextrose

Erythritol

Glucose

Granulated sugar

Guar gum as minor ingredient

Maltodextrin as minor ingredient

"Processed in a facility that also handles"

Raw sugar

Saccharine

Splenda

Sucrose

Vinegar

Wheat starch

Whey protein isolate

Not allowed—avoid:

Bulgur wheat

Brown sugar

Crystalline fructose

Dry milk solids

Fructo-oligosaccharides/FOS

Fructose

Fructose solids

Fruit-juice concentrates (any type)

High-fructose corn syrup (HFCS)

Honey

Hydrogenated starch hydrolysates

Inulin

Isomalt

Kamut

Lactitol

Maltitol

Mannitol

Miso

Modified starch

Molasses

Polydextrose

Sorbitol

Soy protein isolate

Spelt

Sprouted wheat

Texturized vegetable protein

Tomato paste

Wheat berries

Wheat flour, enriched

Wheat flour, all purpose

Wheat flour, white

Wheat flour, whole wheat

Whey protein concentrate

Xylitol

Dining Out Tips

You will find it easier to prepare your food at home while on the diet. At home, you have full control over ingredients used in recipes. You can read the food labels for all prepared foods on your menus. At restaurants, this will not be as easy. If you do have to dine out, order the simplest possible food preparations, with all ingredients clearly visible. Question the wait staff or the cook to find out whether there may be hidden ingredients that are not allowed for you.

Breakfast ideas at restaurants:

- Oatmeal (prepared with water) and a small banana

- Fried, hard-boiled or scrambled eggs (prepared with water), hash brown potatoes or grits and 1/3 cup orange juice

Lunch or dinner ideas at restaurants:

- Salad with allowed vegetables and meats; oil and vinegar applied at the table

- At an Asian restaurant, rice or rice noodles with steamed or sautéed allowed vegetables and meat; no breading, no sauce

- At an Indian restaurant, rice with tandoori chicken

- At a Mexican restaurant, chicken or beef enchilada or fajitas, made with corn tortillas, no cheese or pieces of onion or garlic

Symptom Rating Worksheet

Date: _____

This week's challenge or elimination, if any:

_____

	Day 1	Day 2	Day 3	Day 4	Day 5	Day 6	Day 7	Sum
Diarrhea								
Urgency								
Constipation								
Pain/cramps								
Bloating								
Gas								

Rate the impact of the symptoms on a scale of 0-3:

0=no or transient symptoms

1=mild; occasional episodes of short duration

2=moderate; frequent episodes of prolonged discomfort interfering with some social activities or work (for urgency, 2=frequent sudden need for toilet)

3=severe; prolonged episodes with only transient relief, seriously interfering with social performance or work (for urgency, 3=unable to control bowels)

For "diarrhea" note the total number of bowel movements for the entire 24-hour period.

At the end of the week, add up your score for each symptom and write the number in the column marked, "Sum."

Comments:

Symptom Rating Worksheet

Date: _____
This week's challenge or elimination, if any:

_____

	Day 1	Day 2	Day 3	Day 4	Day 5	Day 6	Day 7	Sum
Diarrhea								
Urgency								
Constipation								
Pain/cramps								
Bloating								
Gas								

Rate the impact of the symptoms on a scale of 0-3:

0=no or transient symptoms

1=mild; occasional episodes of short duration

2=moderate; frequent episodes of prolonged discomfort interfering with some social activities or work (for urgency, 2=frequent sudden need for toilet)

3=severe; prolonged episodes with only transient relief, seriously interfering with social performance or work (for urgency, 3=unable to control bowels)

For "diarrhea" note the total number of bowel movements for the entire 24-hour period.

At the end of the week, add up your score for each symptom and write the number in the column marked, "Sum."

Comments:

Symptom Rating Worksheet

Date: _____

This week's challenge or elimination, if any:

_____

	Day 1	Day 2	Day 3	Day 4	Day 5	Day 6	Day 7	Sum
Diarrhea								
Urgency								
Constipation								
Pain/cramps								
Bloating								
Gas								

Rate the impact of the symptoms on a scale of 0-3:

0=no or transient symptoms

1=mild; occasional episodes of short duration

2=moderate; frequent episodes of prolonged discomfort interfering with some social activities or work (for urgency, 2=frequent sudden need for toilet)

3=severe; prolonged episodes with only transient relief, seriously interfering with social performance or work (for urgency, 3=unable to control bowels)

For "diarrhea" note the total number of bowel movements for the entire 24-hour period.

At the end of the week, add up your score for each symptom and write the number in the column marked, "Sum."

Comments:

Symptom Rating Worksheet

Date: _____
This week's challenge or elimination, if any:

_____

	Day 1	Day 2	Day 3	Day 4	Day 5	Day 6	Day 7	Sum
Diarrhea								
Urgency								
Constipation								
Pain/cramps								
Bloating								
Gas								

Rate the impact of the symptoms on a scale of 0-3:

0=no or transient symptoms

1=mild; occasional episodes of short duration

2=moderate; frequent episodes of prolonged discomfort interfering with some social activities or work (for urgency, 2=frequent sudden need for toilet)

3=severe; prolonged episodes with only transient relief, seriously interfering with social performance or work (for urgency, 3=unable to control bowels)

For "diarrhea" note the total number of bowel movements for the entire 24-hour period.

At the end of the week, add up your score for each symptom and write the number in the column marked, "Sum."

Comments:

Symptom Rating Worksheet

Date: _____

This week's challenge or elimination, if any:

_____

	Day 1	Day 2	Day 3	Day 4	Day 5	Day 6	Day 7	Sum
Diarrhea								
Urgency								
Constipation								
Pain/cramps								
Bloating								
Gas								

Rate the impact of the symptoms on a scale of 0-3:

0=no or transient symptoms

1=mild; occasional episodes of short duration

2=moderate; frequent episodes of prolonged discomfort interfering with some social activities or work (for urgency, 2=frequent sudden need for toilet)

3=severe; prolonged episodes with only transient relief, seriously interfering with social performance or work (for urgency, 3=unable to control bowels)

For "diarrhea" note the total number of bowel movements for the entire 24-hour period.

At the end of the week, add up your score for each symptom and write the number in the column marked, "Sum."

Comments:

Symptom Rating Worksheet

Date: _____

This week's challenge or elimination, if any:

	Day 1	Day 2	Day 3	Day 4	Day 5	Day 6	Day 7	Sum
Diarrhea								
Urgency								
Constipation								
Pain/cramps								
Bloating								
Gas								

Rate the impact of the symptoms on a scale of 0-3:

0=no or transient symptoms

1=mild; occasional episodes of short duration

2=moderate; frequent episodes of prolonged discomfort interfering with some social activities or work (for urgency, 2=frequent sudden need for toilet)

3=severe; prolonged episodes with only transient relief, seriously interfering with social performance or work (for urgency, 3=unable to control bowels)

For "diarrhea" note the total number of bowel movements for the entire 24-hour period.

At the end of the week, add up your score for each symptom and write the number in the column marked, "Sum."

Comments:

Symptom Rating Worksheet

Date: _____

This week's challenge or elimination, if any:

_____

	Day 1	Day 2	Day 3	Day 4	Day 5	Day 6	Day 7	Sum
Diarrhea								
Urgency								
Constipation								
Pain/cramps								
Bloating								
Gas								

Rate the impact of the symptoms on a scale of 0-3:

0=no or transient symptoms

1=mild; occasional episodes of short duration

2=moderate; frequent episodes of prolonged discomfort interfering with some social activities or work (for urgency, 2=frequent sudden need for toilet)

3=severe; prolonged episodes with only transient relief, seriously interfering with social performance or work (for urgency, 3=unable to control bowels)

For "diarrhea" note the total number of bowel movements for the entire 24-hour period.

At the end of the week, add up your score for each symptom and write the number in the column marked, "Sum."

Comments:

Symptom Rating Worksheet

Date: _____

This week's challenge or elimination, if any:

_____

	Day 1	Day 2	Day 3	Day 4	Day 5	Day 6	Day 7	Sum
Diarrhea								
Urgency								
Constipation								
Pain/cramps								
Bloating								
Gas								

Rate the impact of the symptoms on a scale of 0-3:

0=no or transient symptoms

1=mild; occasional episodes of short duration

2=moderate; frequent episodes of prolonged discomfort interfering with some social activities or work (for urgency, 2=frequent sudden need for toilet)

3=severe; prolonged episodes with only transient relief, seriously interfering with social performance or work (for urgency, 3=unable to control bowels)

For "diarrhea" note the total number of bowel movements for the entire 24-hour period.

At the end of the week, add up your score for each symptom and write the number in the column marked, "Sum."

Comments:

Symptom Rating Worksheet

Date: _____

This week's challenge or elimination, if any:

_____

	Day 1	Day 2	Day 3	Day 4	Day 5	Day 6	Day 7	Sum
Diarrhea								
Urgency								
Constipation								
Pain/cramps								
Bloating								
Gas								

Rate the impact of the symptoms on a scale of 0-3:

0=no or transient symptoms

1=mild; occasional episodes of short duration

2=moderate; frequent episodes of prolonged discomfort interfering with some social activities or work (for urgency, 2=frequent sudden need for toilet)

3=severe; prolonged episodes with only transient relief, seriously interfering with social performance or work (for urgency, 3=unable to control bowels)

For "diarrhea" note the total number of bowel movements for the entire 24-hour period.

At the end of the week, add up your score for each symptom and write the number in the column marked, "Sum."

Comments:

Symptom Rating Worksheet

Date: _____

This week's challenge or elimination, if any:

_____

	Day 1	Day 2	Day 3	Day 4	Day 5	Day 6	Day 7	Sum
Diarrhea								
Urgency								
Constipation								
Pain/cramps								
Bloating								
Gas								

Rate the impact of the symptoms on a scale of 0-3:

0=no or transient symptoms

1=mild; occasional episodes of short duration

2=moderate; frequent episodes of prolonged discomfort interfering with some social activities or work (for urgency, 2=frequent sudden need for toilet)

3=severe; prolonged episodes with only transient relief, seriously interfering with social performance or work (for urgency, 3=unable to control bowels)

For "diarrhea" note the total number of bowel movements for the entire 24-hour period.

At the end of the week, add up your score for each symptom and write the number in the column marked, "Sum."

Comments:

Index

T

U

V

W

X

Y

About the Author

PATSY DANEHY CATSOS is a registered, licensed dietitian in private practice in Portland, Maine. Ms. Catsos specializes in medical nutrition therapy for gastrointestinal diseases and disorders. She has a personal and a professional interest in this field, since she herself has ulcerative colitis. Ms. Catsos is an adjunct faculty member at Andover College in Portland. She is a freelancer for the food and nutrition forum of *www.RaisingMaine.com*. Ms. Catsos is a member of the American Dietetic Association and a board member of the Maine Dietetic Association.

Ms. Catsos has a bachelor's degree in Nutritional Science from Cornell University. In 1985 she completed a combined internship and a master's degree program at Boston University and Beth Israel Hospital in Boston, Massachusetts. She then worked for several years as a research dietitian and nutrient database manager at Tufts University School of Medicine. Ms. Catsos is the author or co-author of a number of published articles and peer-reviewed research papers. In 2005, she resumed her dietetics practice, and sees clients at Nutrition Works, LLC in Portland, Maine (*www.nutritionworks.us*). Married since 1984 to Paul Catsos, Ms. Catsos has three children and resides in Cape Elizabeth, Maine.

Please visit *www.ibsfree.net* or email Ms. Catsos at patsy-catsos@gmail.com for more information about her medical nutrition therapy practice or to learn how to order additional copies of this book.

Bibliography

1   Barrett JS, Gibson PR. Clinical ramifications of mal-absorption of fructose and other short-chain carbohydrates. *Pract Gastroenterol.* 2007;51–65.

2   Choi YK, Kraft N, Zimmerman B, Jackson M, Rao SSC. Fructose intolerance in IBS and utility of fructose-restricted diet. *J Clin Gastroenterol.* 2008 Mar;42(3):233–238.

3   Fernandez-Bañares F, Rosinach M, Esteve M, Forné M, Espinós JC, Maria Viver J, Sugar malabsorption in functional abdominal bloating: a pilot study on the long-term effect of dietary treatment. *J Clin Nutr.* 2006 Oct; 25(5):824–831.

4   Goldstein R, Braverman D, Stankiewicz H. Carbohy-drate malabsorption and the effect of dietary restriction on symptoms of irritable bowel syndrome and functional bowel complaints. *Israel Med Assoc J.* 2000 Aug;2:583–587.

5   Shepherd SJ, Parker FC, Muir JG, Gibson PR. Dietary triggers of abdominal symptoms in patients with irritable bowel syndrome: randomized placebo-controlled evidence. *Clin Gastroenterol H.* 2008 May;6(7):765–771.

6   Shepherd SJ, Gibson, PR. Fructose malabsorption and symptoms of irritable bowel syndrome: guidelines for effec-tive dietary management. *J Am Diet Assoc.* 2006 Oct;106:1631–1639.

7   Brown, JE. *Nutrition Now*, 5th ed. (Belmont, CA: Thompson Wadsworth, 2008). P. 3–6.

8   American Dietetic Association. Welcome page. 2008 http://www.eatright.org/cps/rde/xchg/ada/hs.xsl/index. html.

9   Barrett JS. Clinical.

10   Hadley SK, Gaarder SM. Treatment of irritable bowel syndrome. *Am Fam Physician.* 2005 Dec;72(12):2501–2506.

11   Thiwan S. Lactose intolerance and small bowel bacterial overgrowth in irritable bowel syndrome. The UNC Center for Functional GI and Motility Disorders. 2008 http://www.med.unc.edu/ibs.

12   Kolfenbach L. The pathophysiology, diagnosis and treatment of IBS. *J Amer Acad Phys Assist.* 2007 Jan;(20)1: 16–20.

13   Thiwan, S. Lactose.

14   Akbar A, Yiangou Y, Facer P, Walters JRF, Anand P, Ghosh S. Increased capsaicin receptor TRPV1-expressing sensory fibres in irritable bowel syndrome and their correlation with abdominal pain. *Gut* 2008;57:923–929.

15   Hadley SK. Treatment.

16   Kolfenfach L. The pathophysiology.

17   Simrén M, Axelsson J, Gillberg R, Abrahamsson H, Svedlund J, Björnsson ES. Quality of life in inflammatory bowel disease in remission: the impact of IBS-like symptoms and associated psychological factors. *Am J Gastroenterol.* 2002 Feb;97(2):389–96.

18   Gearry RB, Irving PM, Nathan DM, Barrett JS, Shepherd SJ, Gibson PR. The effect of reduction of poorly absorbed, highly fermentable short chain carbohydrates (FODMAPs) on the symptoms of patients with inflammatory bowel disease (IBD). J Gastroen Hepatol. 2007;22(supp 3):A292.

19   Nathan DM, Shepherd SJ, Berryman M, Muir JG, Iser JH, Gibson PR. Fructose malabsorption in Crohn's disease: a common contributor to symptoms that benefit from dietary modification. J Gastroen Hepatol. 2005;20(Suppl.):A27.

20   Hadley SK. Treatment.

21   Kolfenfach L. The pathophysiology.

22   Barret JS. Clinical.

23   Barret JS. Clinical.

24   Thiwan, S. Lactose.

25   Christie C, ed. *The Florida Medical Nutrition Therapy Manual*, (Florida Dietetic Association) 2005. P. 4.1–4.2.

26   Beyer PL, Caviar EM, McCallum RW. Fructose intake at current levels in the United States may cause gastrointestinal distress in normal adults. *J Am Diet Assoc.* 2005 Oct;105:1559–1566.

27   Choi YK. Fructose.

28   Fernandez-Bañares. Sugar.

29   Barret JS. Clinical.

30   Chatterjee S, Park S, Low K, Kong Y, Pimentel M. The degree of breath methane production in IBS correlates with the severity of constipation. *Am J Gastroenterol.* 2007 Apr;102(4):837–41.

31   Nucera G, Gabrielli M, Lupascu A, Lauritano EC, Santoliquido A, Cremonini F, Cammarota G., Tondi P, Pola P, Gasbarrini G, Gasbarrini A. Abnormal breath tests to lactose, fructose and sorbitol in irritable bowel syndrome may be explained by small intestinal bacterial overgrowth. *Aliment Pharm Therap.* 2005;21(11):1391–1395.

32   Thiwan, S. Lactose.

33   Signet Diagnostic Corporation. Leap-Disease Management Website. 2008 http://www.nowleap.com/index.html.

34   Shepherd SJ. Fructose.

35   Barret JS. Clinical.

36   Shepherd SJ. Fructose.

37   Lee CY, Shallenberger RS, Vittum MT. Free sugars in fruits and vegetables. *New York's Food and Life Sciences Bulletin*. 1970;1:1–12.

38   Lavender, R. Following the ripening of bananas. *Chem Sci*. 2006 Feb;3 2008 http://www.rsc.org/Publishing/ChemScience/Volume/2006/03/ripening_of_bananas.asp

39   McNeil Nutritionals, Frequently Asked Questions About Lactaid Milk, 2008 http://www.lactaid.com/products/index.jhtml?id=lactaid/products/milkfaq.inc

40   Shepherd SJ. Fructose.

41   Brown, JE. *Nutrition*. P.1–9.

42   Lee CY. *Free*.

43   Food and Agriculture Organization of the United Nations. *Carbohydrates in Human Nutrition*, Report of a Joint FAO/WHO Consultation, Rome. 1997 Apr. 2008 http://www.fao.org/docrep/W8079E/w8079e00.HTM.

44   Barret JS. Clinical.

45   Food and Agriculture Organization of the United Nations. *Carbohydrates*.

46   Barret JS. Clinical.

47   Food and Agriculture Organization of the United Nations. *Carbohydrates*.

48   Niness KR. Inulin and oligogructose: what are they? J Nutr. 1999; 129:1402S–1406S.

49   Stone-Dorshow T, Levitt MD. Gaseous response to ingestion of a poorly absorbed fructo-oligosaccharide sweetener. *Am J Clin Nutr*. 1987;46:61–5.

50   Shepherd SJ. Fructose.

51   Goldstein, R. Carbohydrate.

52   Beyer PL. Fructose.

53   Nucera G. Abnormal.

54   Beyer PL. Fructose.

55   Beyer PL. Fructose.

56   Barret JS. Clinical.

57   American Gastroenterological Association. Lactose Intolerance. 2008 http://www.gastro.org/wmspage. cfm?parm1=854.

58   Christie C, ed. *The Florida*. P. 4.1–4.2.

59   McNeil Nutritionals. Frequently Asked Questions About Lactaid Milk, 2008 http://www.lactaid.com/page. jhtml?id=lactaid/expert/faq1.inc.

60   Barret JS. Clinical.

61   Vos MB, Kimmons JE, Gillespie C, Welsh J, Blanck HM. Dietary fructose consumption among US children and adults: the Third National Health and Nutrition Examination Survey, *Medscape J Med*. 2008;10(7):160 http://www.medscape. com/viewarticle/576945.

62   Bray GA. Consumption.

63   Barret JS. Clinical.

64   ACH Food Companies Inc. Nutritional Facts. 2008 http://www.karosyrup.com/nutrition.asp.

65   Hanover ML, White JS. Manufacturing, composition and applications of fructose. *Am J Clin Nutr.*1993;58(suppl):724S–32S.

66   Bray GA. Consumption.

67   Vos MB. Dietary.

68   Barret JS. Clinical.

69   Barret JS. Clinical.

70   Rumessen, JJ, Gudmand-Høyer E. Fructans of chicory: intestinal transport and fermentation of different chain lengths and relation to fructose and sorbitol malabsorption. *Am J Clin Nutr* 1998;68:357–64.

71   Barret JS. Clinical.

72   Barret JS. Clinical.

73   Moshfegh, AJ, Friday JE, Goldman JP, Chug A, Jaspreet K. Presence of inulin and oligofructose in the diets of Americans, *J Nutr*. 1999;129:1407S–1411S.

74   American Dietetic Association. Polyols: Sweet Benefits. 2008 http://www.eatright.org/ada/files/Polyols_2008.pdf.

75   Health Canada. Sugar alcohols (polyols) and polydextrose used as sweeteners in food. 2005. 2008 http://www.hc-sc.gc.ca/fn-an/securit/addit/sweeten-edulcor/polyols_poly-dextose_factsheet-polyols_polydextose_fiche-eng.php.

76   The Sugar Association, Inc. Sugar. Sweet by Nature. 2008   http://www.sugar.org/consumers/sweet_by_nature. asp?id=278.

77   Arrigoni E, Brouns F, Amadò R. Human gut microbiota does not ferment erythritol. Brit J Nutr. 2005;94:643-646.

78   DeVries J, Post B, Medallian Laboratories. Polydextrose technical bulletin. 2008 http://www.medlabs.com/file. aspx?FileID=107.

79   Health Canada. Sugar.

80   Barret JS. Clinical.

Made in the USA
Lexington, KY
16 June 2011